LISTENING
TO
PAIN

Finding Words, Compassion, and Relief

DAVID BIRO, MD

W. W. NORTON & COMPANY New York • London

Originally published under the title *The Language
of Pain: Finding Words, Compassion, and Relief*

For information about permission to reproduce selections from this book,
write to Permissions, W. W. Norton & Company, Inc.,
500 Fifth Avenue, New York, NY 10110

For information about special discounts for bulk purchases,
please contact W. W. Norton Special Sales at
specialsales@wwnorton.com or 800-233-4830

Manufacturing by RR Donnelley
Book design by JAM Design
Production manager: Louise Mattarelliano

Library of Congress has cataloged the hardcover edition as follows:

Biro, David, 1964–
Listening to pain : finding words, compassion, and relief / David Biro.
    p. cm.
Originally published: Language of pain. New York : W.W. Norton, c2010.
Includes bibliographical references and index.
ISBN 978-0-393-34025-9 (pbk.)
1. Pain—Physiological aspects. 2. Pain—Psychological aspects.
I. Biro, David, 1964– Language of pain. II. Title.
RB127.B54 2011
616'.0472—dc22

                        2011008257

W. W. Norton & Company, Inc.
500 Fifth Avenue, New York, N.Y. 10110
www.wwnorton.com

W. W. Norton & Company Ltd.
Castle House, 75/76 Wells Street, London W1T 3QT

1 2 3 4 5 6 7 8 9 0

More Praise for

LISTENING TO PAIN

"Erudite and ambitious. . . . [*Listening to Pain*] resonate[s] not only with the common certainties of pain and death but also with the infinite individuality of human life and human voice."

—Perri Klass, *Washington Post*

"True genius. . . . Each thoughtfully selected example helps to find the language that Biro seeks. . . . Through many individual components, Biro creates a larger portrait of pain, deftly addressing the physical as well as psychological aspects of the human experience of pain. . . . He moves beyond simply recounting events and instead transforms how the reader thinks about pain."

—Preeti N. Malani, *Journal of the American Medical Association*

"[Biro] explains how those in pain may use metaphor to heal suffering and loneliness when merely descriptive language falls short." —*Booklist*

"Biro is able to bridge the gap between patient and doctor. . . . This well-researched book will be helpful to medical professionals and psychologists as well as those who suffer from chronic or extreme pain, offering encouragement and inspiration for explaining their experiences to their doctors."

—Helena Travka, *Library Journal*

"Here's a pain medication you can't get at the pharmacy. . . . Thoughtful, lyrical. . . . We should pay attention to Biro's difficult, complicated lesson."

—*Publishers Weekly*

"It's amazing that such a big topic hasn't been discussed more. . . . [Biro] does a remarkable job sifting through philosophy and coming up with something very practical."

—James Cottrill,
Headache and Migraine News

"Enlightening . . . rich in its philosophic and literary meditations on pain and metaphor. . . . Biro is to be commended for the acuity and sensitivity of his reflections on the patient's experience in this thoughtful and richly referenced book."

—Raymond C. Tait, *PsycCritiques*,
the American Psychological Association

Also by David Biro

One Hundred Days:
My Unexpected Journey
from Doctor to Patient

For Dolores and Laszlo

and

For Daniella, Luca, and Daniel

Contents

Introduction / 11

PART I: THE CRISIS

1: The Quintessential Private Experience / 23

2: The Elusiveness of Pain / 36

3: The Public Side of Pain / 48

4: Man's Puny Inexhaustible Voice / 56

PART II: THE SOLUTION

5: Metaphor and Worldmaking / 65

6: The Weapon / 79

7: Literary Agency / 97

8: The Mirror / 129

9: The X-Ray / 167

Postscript / 213

Notes / 221

References / 235

Acknowledgments / 243

Text Credits / 247

Index / 249

LISTENING
TO
PAIN

Introduction

Neoptolemus:
What is this thing that comes upon you suddenly,
that makes you cry and moan so?

Philoctetes:
Terrible it is, beyond words' reach. But pity me.

—SOPHOCLES, *Philoctetes*

Pain is difficult to express. Language and pain seem as far apart as the opposite poles of an electric current. While language can capture much of the diverse range of human experience, it fails us in the case of pain. We try to find the right words, but typically come up empty. We end up wringing our hands and resigning ourselves to silence. A perfect image of the experience, as Elaine Scarry, our most provocative thinker on the subject, suggests, is Edvard Munch's painting *The Scream*. Munch's figure clutches the sides of his head with his hands. His mouth, open wide, is poised to vocalize his anguish. But no sound is uttered. No one—neither the boaters, nor the two figures walking away, nor viewers of the painting—can hear the man's scream.

This is not an exaggeration. I recognized its truth early on in my medical training, while first observing the awkward interaction between patients and physicians. But it wasn't until years later, when I became a patient myself, that I truly understood Munch's terrifying vision. Shortly after finishing my residency, I was diagnosed with a rare and life-threatening blood disorder. Between the

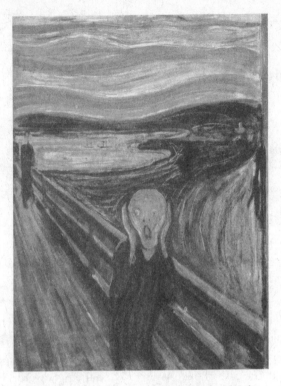

The Scream by Edvard Munch. © 2009 *The Munch Museum / The Munch-Ellingsen Group / Artists Rights Society* (ARS), NY.

physical symptoms (an intermittent ache in one eye and increasing lethargy) and the psychological ones (anger and fear about what was happening and what might happen), I could barely think straight. During visits with the doctor, I stuttered and stammered like a bumbling fool. Still, my inarticulateness paled in comparison with what took place in the hospital during my bone marrow transplant. At its most intense, the pain literally strangled my vocal cords. Silenced, I felt just like Munch's sufferer: wanting to scream as loudly as I could but unable to make a sound.

Expressing pain seems impossible, whether the paralyzing pain from ulcers spreading through the gastrointestinal tract or the less debilitating kind caused by a blood clot in the eye. Patients, even physicians who become patients, find themselves tongue-tied. We hesitate, unsure how to begin—how to describe what feels so immediate and yet so intangible at the same time. When and if we do make the attempt, we're convinced that no one else, especially the person in the white coat at the other end of the examining table, could ever understand.

The medical community is aware of the problem. Over the years it has tried to help patients articulate their pain. One of the most promising attempts was the McGill Pain Questionnaire, created in the 1970s. It provides patients with lengthy lists of descriptive words they can choose to convey their feelings. But with the exception of highly specialized pain clinics, medical practitioners rarely use the questionnaire these days. It may be too complicated to explain. It takes too much time to fill out. And perhaps, despite the good intentions of its authors, both parties remain unsatisfied: doctors are uncomfortable with the form's metaphorical language, and patients want even more of it.

Instead, health-care providers rely much more commonly on the very basic, almost primitive series of pictures known as the Faces Pain Scale:

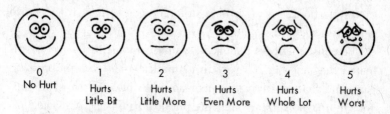

| 0 | 1 | 2 | 3 | 4 | 5 |
| No Hurt | Hurts Little Bit | Hurts Little More | Hurts Even More | Hurts Whole Lot | Hurts Worst |

Wong Baker FACES Pain Rating Scale from Hockenberry, MJ, and Wilson, D: *Wong's Essentials of Pediatric Nursing*, ed. 8, St. Louis, 2009, Mosby. *Used with Permission. Copyright Mosby.*

The scale dispenses with words altogether and focuses on just one aspect of pain: its intensity. Elaine Scarry is right when she says that pain causes us to regress to "a state anterior to language, to the sounds and cries a human being makes before language is learned." In fact no one even bothers to talk anymore in the clinic or emergency room. We simply point to the picture and keep our pain to ourselves.

But we mustn't think the problem is confined to the average person. Even those with a gift for language, our greatest poets and writers, have found it difficult to capture pain in words. Emily Dickinson once wrote that pain "has an Element of Blank." The patients in W. H. Auden's poem "Surgical Ward" live beneath their bandages and no longer communicate in human terms: "It is not talk like ours, but groans they smother." And Virginia Woolf too, that most lyrical of prose writers, found herself at a loss for words in the summer of 1925 during a bout of influenza. So she looked to famous authors of the past to see if they had more to say about such a common part of life. Surprisingly, she found very little. Literature is concerned with the mind, she decided, not the daily dramas of the body. When it came to pain, there was a poverty of language: "Let a sufferer try to describe a pain in his head and language at once runs dry."

The inexpressibility of pain, then, is our starting point. From there, this book has two main goals: to explore the reasons for this inexpressibility and to discover ways of overcoming them. Why does the language run dry, and how can we restore its flow? By answering these questions, I hope to help sufferers recover their voice and to generate a rhetoric of pain.

The consequences of silence are unacceptable. It has been estimated that one out of every five Americans suffers from chronic pain, and that staggering number does not include the many millions more who suffer from acute physical pain or psychological illnesses like depression. If we wish to relieve their pain—and it will be our pain too at some point—we must first hear it. On the most practical level, the medical profession must hear it. Physicians rely on a patient's story—how well he or she is able to describe symptoms—as much as they do on stethoscopes and blood tests. Studies have shown that the more detailed those descriptions are, the better physicians are at pinpointing the source of pain and administering appropriate treatment. Yet most patients tend to be about as inarticulate as I was when it comes to pain, and physicians often either are unable to coax them in the right direction or don't have enough time and patience to try. The result is that both parties quickly become frustrated and fall back on pointing at the sad faces on the chart and writing indiscriminate prescriptions. Even worse, the pain may be ignored, which happens more commonly than the medical profession would like to admit.

But it's not only a matter of responding to the strictly physical demands of pain, of treating the cancer or prescribing the right analgesics. Pain of any variety isolates us from our family and closest friends. No one could feel what I felt during my transplant—not my wife or my parents or my sisters. And the inability to find words for my feelings only exacerbated my loneliness. This too is a consequence of silence, one that extends beyond medicine. Even when the pain of cancer, arthritis, or depression has proven refractory to treatment, language still offers the potential to help. By enabling us to communicate (from the Latin *communicare*, "to share") our feelings, language can replace isolation with community; it can relieve our suffering when chemotherapy or psychotropics cannot. Therefore, it is critical that we work together—physicians, caregivers, patients, and indeed all members of society—to ensure that that this pervasive part of human experience finds a place in our collective vocabulary.

This book is divided into two parts. The first explores pain and its effects on the individual, showing how it rises to the level of crisis, inevitably thrusting us inward to the solitude of personal experience. Pain erects a wall between us and the outside world. At the same time, it prevents us from breaching that wall by communicating the experience to others. Despite its overwhelming presence, pain has the elusive quality of an absence, an absence not only of words to describe it (that is, a linguistic absence) but also of ways to think about it (a conceptual one).

Once we determine the reasons for the crisis, we are in a better position to find a solution. In the second part of the book, we learn that whenever we are confronted with something difficult or impossible to grasp, there is only one way open to us: metaphor. By speaking of what we don't know in terms of what we do know, metaphor replaces absence with presence. It illuminates aspects of existence that would otherwise remain in the dark, from private experiences such as pain and our belief in God to new scientific theories of how the objective world works. In these cases, metaphor isn't merely a rhetorical device that dresses up language but a powerful and necessary resource of the imagination that literally extends the boundaries of our shared world.

From a general way of responding to pain, we move to more specific ones. Three different metaphorical strategies are presented, strategies that draw on three familiar objects: the weapon, the mirror, and the X-ray. By far the most common strategy is what Elaine Scarry calls the language of agency. Here sufferers imagine an agent that moves against and injures the body. This type of metaphor is used when patients talk of pain as stabbing or shooting. A second strategy occurs when pain is projected onto other objects, from other people to nonhuman objects in our environment, like animals and trees. Projection metaphors enable sufferers to validate and better understand their pain. In the third strategy, people create images of the inside of the body with words, what we will call anatomic metaphors. Peering underneath the skin, so to speak, sufferers imagine a source for their sensations. Common to these strategies is the desire to replace what is inside and inaccessible with what is outside and directly perceptible.

As we follow the thread of the argument, it will become apparent that pain, as distressing a part of life as it is, provides us with an extraordinary opportunity. A moment of extremity, pain urges us to take extreme measures to respond and express ourselves. By forging novel ways to think and speak through metaphor, we ordinary people become creators, not very different from artists like Edvard Munch, Emily Dickinson, and Virginia Woolf. Conversely, those on the outside, present at such moments, are witnesses to a kind of birthing point of language.

The sources for this work are the words of actual patients and accounts of pain found in literature. Real words from real people offer the advantage of authenticity and are therefore extremely compelling. But the stories of suffering imagined by our best writers have as much to offer in building a rhetoric of pain; in a sense, the artificially constructed world of literature (or any art form, for that matter, such as the paintings of Edvard Munch and Frida Kahlo) can be more "real" than the real one. During times of crisis, we see from only one perspective and events go by quickly, barely giving us the opportunity to respond in meaningful ways. Art affords us the luxury of seeing from multiple perspectives and in a less hectic time frame. It enables us to *see* and then reflect, thereby representing our reality more fully and accurately.

A second reason for drawing on literary accounts has to do with the intrinsic difficulties of expressing pain. It is precisely when language fails—when we are in love, for example, or when we find ourselves in the midst of beauty or pain—that we turn to our greatest artists for help. The truth is that most of us don't possess the resources to respond as articulately as we might wish at such moments. Who better to learn from than those who possess a talent for expression and have dedicated their lives to refining it?

The downside of using literature, however, is its lack of practicality. What use, we might ask, is the language of Dickinson and Woolf to the man in the street? What use are their extraordinary yet rarified metaphors—James Joyce's description of an earache in terms of the roar and stop of a train as it goes through a tunnel or Tolstoy's projecton of his character's pain onto trees in the Russian wilderness? Real people don't talk like that, and if they did, physicians would most likely order a psychiatric consultation. But the point is not to mimic the words of great artists. Rather, it is to see them in the range of the possible, as reflecting an ideal of sorts. We don't necessarily have to talk like Tolstoy or Joyce to realize and draw on the potential shapes and patterns words can take.

In this work I speak about pain as if it were a single well-circumscribed entity, even though this is clearly not the case. As Alphonse Daudet, a nineteenth-century novelist and patient, once wrote in his memoir, *In the Land of Pain*:

> [There is] no general theory about pain. Each patient discovers his own, and the nature of pain varies, like a singer's voice, according to the acoustics of the hall.

Daudet, who suffered from tertiary syphilis, rightly points to the variety of experience that falls under the heading of pain. There is acute pain and chronic pain, physical pain and psychological pain, and varying mixtures of the above (for example, the psychological aspects of physical pain). People experience pain differently, and the same person may experience pain differently on different occasions (depending on the "acoustics," or context). We also know that people of different cultures ascribe different meanings to pain, and that in some instances pain can actually be viewed in a positive light.

Yet despite this variety, I argue that there is a common underlying structure. Most simply defined, pain is an all-consuming internal experience that threatens to destroy everything except itself—family, friends, language, the world, one's thoughts, and ultimately even one's self. In pain, as Munch's sufferer screams to us from the canvas, *there is nothing but the pain*. Understood in this way, while the intensity and character of pain may vary, its essence remains constant. Patients with chronic illnesses, for example, develop ways to deal with their day-to-day pain until it flares up and becomes all-consuming again, instantly obliterating their coping mechanisms along with everything else. The same holds true for the psychological pain of depression or grief. While it may differ qualitatively from the pain of shingles or migraine, it is indistinguishable in terms of its world- and self-negating potential. At times, in fact, psychological pain may surpass—may even be *more painful than*—some of its physical counterparts. That is why the experiences of William Styron (*Darkness Visible*) and Joan Didion (*The Year of Magical Think-*

ing) are just as relevant to this work as those of Alphonse Daudet and so many others who suffer from physical illnesses.

Furthermore, while the issue of pain's inexpressibility is a practical one with practical implications—everybody at some point experiences pain and needs help communicating it to doctors and family—it also raises some very complicated questions. The quintessential private experience, pain underscores our separateness from other people. Can we really convey our subjective experiences to another person? Can other people ever understand how we feel? Or are disconnection and isolation just facts of the human condition? If, however, it were possible to communicate pain, what form would it take? How might language, which is only meaningful if we can share it with others, gain traction in so private and personal a sphere?

These are important questions, and I discuss the work of philosophers such as Maurice Merleau-Ponty, Ludwig Wittgenstein, and Nelson Goodman, who have wrestled with them over the years. I try to explain their concepts in the plainest terms, making this work as accessible as possible.

My goal, no doubt, is an idealistic one. While I believe that pain can be represented in language, it is unrealistic to assume that communication is always possible. At its most intense, pain really does consume everything except itself. I began to think about pain and language in medical school and then graduate school—in the abstract, to be sure, since I'd been relatively pain-free until then. When I realized that my education was about to take a practical turn because I had to undergo a bone marrow transplant, I was naively excited about the opportunity. Not to miss documenting a single moment of the pain promised me during my two-month stay in the hospital, I packed pens, paper, computer, and even a tape recorder, just in case I became too weak to write. Yet despite my grandiose plans, when the pain finally struck, I was rendered as mute as Munch's sufferer, despite the constant flow of morphine dripping into my veins. All I wanted to do was to crawl inside a hole and shut my eyes until it, or I, just went away.

There are no words. The truth is that there are no words when one is in severe pain. We are entirely isolated from others at these moments. It is only afterward—hours, days, weeks, and in some cases years afterward—that language becomes possible again. In one of his more cynical moments, Daudet questions whether words have any use at all in describing what pain feels like: "Words only come when everything is over, when things have calmed down. They refer only to memory and are either powerless or untruthful."

While I agree with Daudet that pain destroys language, I don't believe it destroys the desire for language. Nor do I believe that the words which come later are powerless or untruthful. On the contrary, those words are of vital importance. Pain isn't always so intense; it tends to ebb and flow, as do our awareness and responses to it. And while language may be impossible for those situated at pain's peaks, it is not so for those residing in its valleys, when the pain lets up and we recover our breath. At these moments sufferers desperately want to escape from their holes, the silence and loneliness, and return to the world we share with others. Joan Didion felt this desire some nine months after her husband died, when she began writing *The Year of Magical Thinking*. Even Alphonse Daudet, despite his reservations, went on to describe his pain, and in the most eloquent terms. Many others too have felt compelled to fill the void opened up by pain in whatever way they could, whether by writing, confiding to other patients in support groups, or communicating on Internet chat rooms. At these moments, language, the means of expression we are most comfortable with, becomes truly therapeutic—a form of medicine that has the power to relieve our suffering.

PART I

THE
CRISIS

1

The Quintessential Private Experience

> Indeed, the most intense feeling we know of, to the point of blotting out other experiences, namely, the experience of great pain, is at the same time the most private and least communicable of all.
>
> —Hannah Arendt, *The Human Condition*

Harry lies on a cot at the foot of Mount Kilimanjaro. An infection in his leg has progressed to gangrene, and the wound looks and smells awful. His girlfriend tries to comfort him but is not very successful. This is partly because of a lack of understanding—she comes from a different social class. But even if the two were better suited, it is clear that at least in this particular instance, there is little chance for meaningful communication.

Illness has radically transformed Harry's perspective. Before, life went on in the outside world—he worked, he played, he drank, he made love. Now everything important is taking place inside his body. In the early stages of the infection, Harry suffered a great deal of pain. But the pain is on the wane now, and in its place is a numbness that is even more distressing. Because of the wall between them, his girlfriend perceives none of this.

Isolated, Harry tries to make sense of what is happening to him. He can clearly see the wound creeping up his leg but has difficulty determining what it means for him. How bad is the infection? Could it spread further? Will he die? He desperately wishes his girlfriend—someone, anyone—could help answer these questions. He asks her over and over again, telling her he fears the worst. No, no, she answers, everything will be all right.

But Harry has his doubts, because of the strange sensations that continue to come and go—strange because while undoubtedly real, they are vague and indeterminate. What is happening? Is it a new pain? Is he just reacting to the smell of the wound? Is it because he's close to death? Or perhaps a combination of all three? Regardless of how he interprets them, the sensations consume him. And when they are most intense, he asks his girlfriend whether she feels them too. No, she tells him, she feels nothing.

"I do," he says.

> He had just felt death come by again . . . death had come and rested its head on the foot of the cot and he could smell its breath . . . [Death] can have a wide snout like a hyena.

Harry's connection to the world has been severed. He has retreated into the depths of his body, the only world that matters now. His girlfriend cannot penetrate that world; what is so overwhelmingly present for him is entirely absent for her. Nor can he convey what is happening inside him; language has become useless. Harry is alone.

PAIN FROM THE INSIDE

Harry is not a real person. He is a character in Ernest Hemingway's story "The Snows of Kilimanjaro." But he experiences the isolation of real people who are ill and in pain.

When I was in the hospital, although I was surrounded by the people I loved most—my wife, parents, sisters—I felt completely detached. The only thing in the world that mattered was what was happening inside my body—the disease in my bone marrow, its response to chemotherapy and radiation, *my* response to chemotherapy and radiation. And those events, unlike the upcoming presidential election between Clinton and Dole or the snow falling outside the window, were completely unknowable and unfeelable for my family. As close as they were to me, they might as well have been on another planet. Like most patients, I felt like Hemingway's Harry, and perhaps even more like the French journalist Jean-Dominique Bauby. After a stroke left him completely paralyzed, he imagined himself imprisoned in an old-fashioned diving bell suspended in the ocean depths, sinking farther and farther away from his family and friends. This is where pain sends us.

The basis for this sense of detachment is a radical shift in perspective. Ordinarily we are social beings, constantly turning outward to face the world, which is why the phenomenologists, a loosely knit group of twentieth-century philosophers, spoke of our lived existence as a *being-in-the-world*. In many ways this is obvious. We literally face outward—our eyes, ears, nose, and tongue point us toward the people and objects in our environment. And it's not merely a matter of specific sensory organs or body parts. Our bodies as a whole continually push us into the world, when we walk and talk, when we eat and drink, when we work and play.

More important, though perhaps less intuitive, this same orientation holds true for our inner life. Just like our actions and perceptions, our emotions and thoughts reach toward external objects and people. We dream of material *success*, get angry with our *children*, think about our next *meal*, fall in love with a beautiful *person*. True, the dream, the anger, the thoughts, and the falling in love are deeply personal and subjective. Other people can't experience them and know precisely how we feel, which can make us feel disconnected. Still, because the dreaming and thinking and loving are directed to things and people in the external world, because they are about or refer to objects other than ourselves, they reflect our extroversion. Our natural perspective, so fundamentally outward-facing, works to ensure that we are always vitally connected to the community at large.

Illness, particularly pain, changes this perspective. We turn inward and retract like mollusks. Our network of connections with the world—our speech and actions, thoughts and feelings—begins to disintegrate. Everything seems irrelevant and superfluous, everything except what is happening inside us: the pain and other odd sensations. These sensations are unlike other internal experiences, for they do not point to the world beyond us. In fact, they don't seem to point anywhere except, self-reflexively, to themselves; when we are in pain, there's nothing but the pain. Nor do we believe we can ever share this all-consuming, all-important experience with another person. Other people, like Harry's girlfriend or my wife and parents, as well-intentioned as they might be, can never understand. All of which makes us feel more and more like Bauby's lonely deep-sea diver, slipping farther into the cold, dark depths.

Because of this radical shift in perspective, the experiences of illness and pain call to mind another phenomenological concept. The *epoché*, literally a "suspension," was conceived as a thought experiment that could be used to corroborate the notion of lived existence as a being-in-the-world. Can we imagine, the phenomenologists asked rhetorically, suspending our ties with other people and the world, putting them "out of play"? Is it possible to focus solely on the privacy of our self without any outside interference? The answer is unequivocally no, except perhaps in very small doses and in limited settings—during meditation, for example, or intense physical activity. Such detachment is difficult to sustain. How long can we think without thinking of something? How long can we concentrate on the body before looking beyond it to the person standing in front of us? Not very long. A strictly solitary existence is impossible even to imagine.

It is because we are through and through compounded of relationships with the world that for us the only way to become aware of the fact is to suspend the resultant activity . . . to put it "out of play." . . . Reflection does not withdraw from the world towards the unity of consciousness as the world's basis . . . it slackens the intentional threads which attach us to the world and thus brings them to our notice.

The impossibility of imagining an epoché is proof of our connectedness. But the phenomenologists missed an opportunity here, for we don't need a philosophical thought experiment to see that this is true. Pain is a real-life example, and anyone who has experienced pain can tell you so. By its very nature, it threatens to exile us from the world. Moreover, pain is a routine and inescapable part of life, not something we choose or have control over as we do with meditation or sport. And last, because the suspension threatened by pain is so distressing (even more distressing at times than the physical sensation of pain), we can't help but resist it. Sufferers like Munch, Styron, and so many others who are able to express their feelings powerfully demonstrate our commitment to finding a way back to the world.

Even if the epoché of pain isn't necessarily absolute, we mustn't ignore the tendency of those who are ill and in pain *to feel as if it were*, to believe that they are completely detached from the outside world. We can observe this tendency over and over again in literary depictions of illness. Sophocles places the Greek warrior Philoctetes and his festering wound on an isolated island where no one can hear his cries of pain. Alexander Solzhenitsyn envisions a more figurative barrier separating Pavel, the sick protagonist in his novel *Cancer Ward*, from family and friends:

But the harmonious, exemplary Rusanov family, their well-adjusted way of life and their immaculate apartment—in the space of a few days all this had been cut off from him. It was now on the *other* side of his tumor. They were alive and would go on living, whatever happened to their father. However much they might worry, fuss or weep, the tumor was growing like a wall behind him, and on his side of it he was alone.

For Auden, pain radically contracts one's existence to life beneath the bandage. As a result, patients in his poem "Surgical Ward" become so isolated that they seem as remote as the flower arrangements by their beds:

> They are and suffer; that is all they do;
> A bandage hides the place where each is living,
> His knowledge of the world restricted to
> The treatments that the instruments are giving
>
> And lie apart like epochs from each other
> —Truth in their sense is how much they can bear;
> It is not talk like ours, but groans they smother—
> And are remote as plants.

The same sense of detachment is regularly experienced in the hospital rooms of real patients and in the works of nonfiction that such patients have written. Almost a century ago, while suffering from influenza, Virginia Woolf wrote an essay, "On Being Ill," from her sickbed. What struck her most at the time was how apart she felt, the symbolic distance even greater than the actual one:

> How the world has changed its shape; the tools of business grown remote; the sounds of festival become romantic like a merry-go-round heard across far fields; and friends have changed . . . while the whole landscape of life lies remote and fair, like the shore seen from a ship far out at sea.

More recently, the physician Oliver Sacks fell on a mountain in Norway, severely damaging his leg. In great pain, unable to move, and with no one around to help him, Sacks feared he would die. In his memoir, *A Leg to Stand On*, he writes that the "aloneness" he felt at that moment on the mountaintop was "almost sadder than death." Yet it would get even worse for Sacks *after* he was rescued and placed under the care of doctors and nurses at the local hospital:

> I became all of a sudden desolate and deserted, and felt—for the first time, perhaps, since I had entered the hospital—the essential aloneness of the patient, a sort of solitude which I hadn't felt on the mountain.

Although the surgeons were able to repair the damage, Sacks developed an uncommon neurological syndrome in which his leg no longer felt like part of his body. But only he could experience the fear and horror of this unexpected turn of events.

In his memoir, *Darkness Visible*, the novelist William Styron similarly recalled the "ferocious inwardness" that accompanied the pain of depression. About to receive a prestigious literary award at a ceremony in Paris, Styron suddenly found himself recoiling from all the things he had once loved—food, laughter, and language:

> And zombielike, halfway through the dinner, I lost the del Duca prize check . . . and its loss dovetailed well with the other failures of the dinner: my failure to have an appetite for the *grand plateau de fruits de mer* placed before me, failure of even forced laughter and, at last, my virtually total failure of speech. At this point the ferocious *inwardness* of the pain produced an immense distraction that prevented my articulating words beyond a hoarse murmur; I sensed myself turning wall-eyed, monosyllabic. . . . Then, while I was riding in the car, I thought of [the writers] Albert Camus and Romain Gary.

The pain and resulting suspension became so intense that Styron contemplated suicide—the exit strategy used by two of his friends and the ultimate epoché from the world.

PAIN FROM THE OUTSIDE

From the perspective of the sufferer, whether fictional (Harry and Pavel) or real (Woolf, Sacks, and Styron), illness and especially pain give rise to a wall that separates a person from the world. But does this feeling of isolation have any grounding in reality, or is it more a state of mind?

The truth is that the world turns away from the sufferer just as consistently as the sufferer turns away from the world. Consider how society treats the ill—not so differently, as it happens, from the ancient Greeks. We label them sick, dress them in special clothes, and place them in hospitals, nursing homes, and hospices. Moreover, the isolation continues in a more figurative sense in the way we respond or, more accurately, in the way we fail to respond to sufferers. Observers of pain, in fact, have as strong a sense of the pain wall as the sufferer. No matter how much she tries, Harry's girlfriend can't enter the interior and private realm of his sensations. Similarly, my family couldn't experience what I did, which is why they not only seemed to be on a different planet but also acted as if they were. Hovering around my hospital bed, wanting to do something, anything, to comfort me, my wife and family moved with the blankest and most helpless expressions on their faces. *What is happening to my husband, my son, my brother?* they wanted to know. *What can we do to help?* There were no answers to these questions, no way to close the rift that had suddenly opened up between us. And if they couldn't know how I felt, what was there to talk about? We might as well be speaking different languages.

Michael Greenberg confronted the pain wall when his fifteen-year-old daughter became severely ill with bipolar disorder. Recalling those "fable-like days" many years later in his memoir, *Hurry Down Sunshine*, Greenberg writes that he woke up one morning and no longer recognized Sally; every point of connection between them had suddenly vanished.

With each question I await a response, the slightest inclination that whatever spell she is under has broken and she is the child I know again. Each time, however, her otherness is reaffirmed. It is as if the real Sally has been kidnapped and here in her place is a demon, like Solomon's, who has appropriated her body. The ancient superstition of possession! How else to come to grips with this grotesque transformation?

In the most profound sense, Sally and I are strangers; we have no common language.

Despite Sally's pressing need to communicate ("so powerful it's tormenting her") and to feel understood (as strong as her "need for air"), her own father can neither hear nor know her.

Styron remembers how distressing this disconnection was during his illness. Outsiders, even family members and close friends, couldn't relate to him any better than he could relate to them; healthy people just couldn't "imagine a form of torment so alien to everyday experience." Ironically, Styron himself (when pain-free) had once been equally insensitive to friends who were battling depression:

> Romain told me that Jean was being treated for the disorder that afflicted him . . . but none of this registered very strongly, and also meant little. This memory of my relative indifference is important because such indifference demonstrates powerfully the outsider's inability to grasp the essence of the illness. Camus' depression and now Romain Gary's—and certainly Jean's—were abstract ailments to me, in spite of my sympathy, and I hadn't an inkling of its true contours or the nature of the pain so many victims experience as the mind continues its insidious meltdown.

Illness and pain, we might say, emphasize and exaggerate the boundaries between people. They erect a barrier that seems unbreachable from both sides; the barrier separates the sufferer from the world and at the same time the world from the sufferer. This complementarity is brilliantly captured in Auden's poem. The first half of the poem describes the sufferer's withdrawal—"A bandage hides the place where each is living." The second half is a mirror image, textually as well as thematically, of the world withdrawing from the sufferer:

> we stand elsewhere.
>
> For who when healthy can become a foot?
> Even a scratch we can't recall when cured,
> But are boisterous in a moment and believe
>
> In the common world of the uninjured, and cannot
> Imagine isolation. Only happiness is shared,
> And anger, and the idea of love.

The healthy can't see or even imagine what takes place in that invisible space beneath the bandage. The experience, suggests Elaine Scarry, is as remote as some deep subterranean fact, as far away as an intergalactic event.

More formally, pain sets up an ontological divide. There is the reality of the person in pain and the reality of those on the outside. Because there is no way to verify the pain of another, no objective test even in our age of MRIs and PET scans, these radically different realities are unbridgeable. Our only recourse is to take a person at his word—to make the proverbial, and far from reassuring, leap of faith. This brings up another consequence of the pain wall, much more damaging to the sufferer than the aforementioned misunderstandings and miscommunications. Harry's girlfriend, my family, Styron's friends, Auden's uninjured observers—as much as they tried to comprehend the experience of the sufferer, it exceeded the power of their imaginations. But if the realities of the two are so distinct, might not incomprehension lead to skepticism or possibly even outright doubt?

This is precisely what Elaine Scarry argues. Pain generates an ontological divide that puts into question the very existence of pain. From the perspective of the sufferer, there is nothing more real—the experience is the prototype of having certainty (*I am in pain, therefore I exist*). But for the observer, it is the exact opposite. The pain is so remote, it becomes unreal:

> For the person whose pain it is, it is "effortlessly" grasped (that is, even with the most heroic effort, it cannot *not* be grasped); while for the person outside the sufferer's body, what is "effortless" is *not* grasping it (it is easy to remain wholly unaware of its existence; even with effort, one may remain in doubt about its existence or retain the astonishing freedom of denying its existence).

Remember how upset Harry is because his girlfriend can't validate what he is feeling. *How can it be?* he asks. *How can what is so overwhelmingly present for me be so overwhelmingly absent for you?* Yet how much more distressing it would be if Harry's girlfriend went a step further and questioned his sensations, or further still and denied their existence. For the denial would be a denial of Harry himself, since his sensations and his existence have become indistinguishable.

Can Elaine Scarry be right? It's one thing to speak, like Auden and Styron, of the incomprehension of observers, which suggests a kind of passive acceptance of pain's privacy and inaccessibility. But do other people actually doubt and on occasion even dismiss one's pain? Unfortunately, yes. This does indeed happen, and happens more frequently than we might like to believe.

Recently, at the Kings County Hospital emergency room in Brooklyn, a black man came in complaining of pain in his right knee. He was thirty-four years old, shabbily dressed, and gave a history of sickle cell anemia. When he lifted his pants to show where it hurt, there was no swelling or redness, only a slight tenderness to the touch. The young white doctor, a resident, who had never met the man before, tried to reconcile the discrepancy between the exam and the patient's symptoms. After spotting what looked like track marks on the patient's arm, his mind was made up. There was no need to order any further tests (which would have revealed the sickle cell disease–related problem missed on the exam). The patient was faking. He was just another junkie looking for a fix.

Of course we could rationalize the disconnect between the person in pain and the outside observer in this case (as we did in the Hemingway story) by pointing to their obvious differences—race, socio-economic status, and so on. But the same disconnection could easily happen when two people are more like-minded.

Patients of mine—we'll call them Sandy and Eric—grew up together in the suburbs of Philadelphia. They have three children and a great marriage. Sandy has severe rheumatoid arthritis, and Eric is as understanding as a husband can be. But every now and then, he's not so sure about her pain. The other night Sandy woke up after midnight complaining of pain in her wrist. *It really hurts*, she tells Eric. *But you took two Percosets before bed*, he reminds her. She takes a third one and an hour later wakes up again, clutching her wrist. Eric took a Percoset once when he sprained an ankle, and it practically put him into a coma. He can't understand how Sandy can still feel pain after three of them, no matter how bad the injury. He tries to reassure his wife, but it's obvious from the way he looks at her that he has his doubts. Eric goes back to sleep. Sandy stays up most of the night.

One doesn't need to rely on a physician's personal anecdotes to demonstrate people's tendency toward skepticism when observing pain. In the 1970s, researchers began to investigate how well physicians responded to the pain of cancer patients. Specifically, they wanted to find out whether adequate doses of pain medication were being administered. The results of the study were unexpected and embarrassing, to say the least. It turned out that more often than not, physicians did *not* prescribe enough medication. In fact, they consistently undertreated their patients' pain. Now these physicians, let's not forget, were men and women who had been trained and had subsequently accumulated years of experience in caring for sick people. Of course no one believes the physicians were acting maliciously. They had their reasons, the most prominent of which was a fear of causing addiction. But surely they must also have been thinking along the same lines as Eric: *Hmm, that was a whole lot of medicine we gave Mr. X . . . how could he possibly still be in pain?*

Even more troubling than these initial reports is the fact that decades later, nothing had changed. In 1994 the U.S. Department of Health and Human Services revisited the issue by carrying out a similar series of investigations. Their findings were no different from the earlier ones: more than 50 percent of cancer patients didn't receive adequate analgesia, and about 25 percent of them were estimated to die in severe, unrelieved pain. At this point we can no longer rationalize the behavior of physicians by bringing up the addiction argument. We know that addiction doesn't typically develop when drugs are used to alleviate great pain. So what should we conclude? That we can't train health-care providers to respond to patients more effectively? And if the professionals can't be trained, then what are the odds that the rest of us will do any better?

2

The Elusiveness of Pain

Pain—has an Element of Blank—
It cannot recollect
When it begun—or if there were
A time when it was not—

It has no Future—but itself—
Its infinite contain
Its past—enlightened to perceive
New Periods—of Pain.

—EMILY DICKINSON

George S got into a bad car accident seven years ago. The forty-four-year-old contractor and avid runner fractured multiple bones and ruptured two spinal disks. After several operations, the orthopedic surgeons proudly informed him that they had repaired all the damage and he would be as good as new. They were wrong. True, George was able to walk and work again, even run on occasion. But he couldn't sustain the activities for long, because an incapacitating pain would always intervene—one that wound around his back and shot down his legs, freezing him in his tracks.

For a while his doctors were sympathetic. They listened to his complaints and tried to decipher the problem. But when all the tests came back negative and exploratory surgery located no source of the pain, they threw up their hands in frustration. George became even more frustrated. He stopped trying to describe how he felt to the doctors, who were no longer listening and were pushing him out the door with prescriptions for sleeping pills and anxiety medications. In fact, he stopped talking in general, even to his wife and children. He shut himself off and soon became clinically depressed—a new problem and a new source of pain to add to the old one.

There are many patients like George. Because they see pain as unsharable and because others reinforce that belief through their actions, they become resigned. Why bother trying to convince friends, relatives, or doctors if they don't believe you? Why bother trying to convey how you feel if no one will understand?

But resigning oneself to suffer alone doesn't necessarily mean that communication is impossible. We need to address the question of whether there is a solid basis for our feelings. Are there substantive reasons for the difficulties we have in expressing pain?

"Pain—has an Element of Blank," writes Emily Dickinson. Her poem suggests that the blankness has both temporal and spatial dimensions—it seems to go on forever and do so in a space that excludes everything but itself. Pain has no borders, no shape, no coordinates. Its elusiveness resists attempts at representation.

George S spends almost every waking minute focused on this amorphous terrain. All he wants to do is to grab his pain with both hands, to see what is causing it and what he can do to get rid of it. But he can't. As close as he is to it, as sure as he is of it, the pain remains a phantom.

In a similar way, Styron stumbled in the dark during his battle with depression. Years later, after he had recovered, he would return to that shadowy realm in the hope that he could define the terrain more clearly, to make the darkness visible for others (as well as for himself). In *Darkness Visible*, Styron vividly recalls the details leading up to his breakdown. It is late October 1985, and he is in Paris. The evening is chilly, the streets are slick, and the neon sign of the Hotel Washington is glowing. The next day he appears at the grand rococo mansion of Simone del Duca, a large, dark-haired woman of queenly manner. She will present him with a prestigious literary award. Unintentionally, he insults his hostess before the ceremony, and he does everything he can to correct the *malentendu*. But to no avail.

With these finely rendered details, Styron brings his readers with him to the brink of disaster. But when the pain strikes, every shred of lucidity disintegrates. Styron balks. He struggles to find words, but the experience is a blur. The words he manages to stumble on are not quite right. The pain, he writes, is close to physical pain. But the next minute he rejects the characterization: no, it's different. The pain, he tries again later, is like suffocating or drowning. No, that's not right either. The fact is, Styron ultimately concedes, the pain is simply "indescribable." It's impossible even to imagine, not only for someone else *but also for himself*.

Like Dickinson and George S, Styron is responding to the paradox at the heart of pain. Pain is so acutely present and immediate that we can't imagine anything more real. This is why Elaine Scarry believes "that 'having pain' may come to be thought of as the most vibrant example of what it is to 'have certainty.'" Yet at the same time pain lacks the concrete form and shape, the palpability, we normally associate with reality. It's much too diffuse and hazy to wrap our mind around and put into words; it is the darkness that confronts George S and William Styron. And this quality also contributes to the paralysis that these sufferers, and almost everyone else, feels in the grip of pain.

Previously we focused on our instinctive tendency to see pain as private and isolating. We hesitate to speak because we believe no one will understand us. Here, however, the problem is not how we see the experience but the experience itself. It is a blur. How can we possibly describe it? How can we even begin? The inexpressibility of pain, then, isn't necessarily due to an inadequacy or fault with language. We may even say it precedes language. It is the experience and our ability to apprehend it that are problematic. What could we say about something so insubstantial?

The question we grapple with in this chapter is why pain, "so incontestably and unnegotiably present," in Scarry's words, is at the same time so vague and indeterminate. What is it about pain that makes it unique in the spectrum of human experience? What makes it different from other experiences—love, for example, which, while often subjective and blurry, seems more receptive to language? "The merest schoolgirl, when she falls in love," Virginia Woolf tells us, "has Shakespeare or Keats to speak her mind for her; but let a sufferer try to describe a pain in his head and language at once runs dry."

LACK OF INTENTIONALITY

There are two fundamental reasons for the elusiveness of pain: its lack of intentionality, on the one hand, and its inaccessibility as a bodily event, on the other. Earlier we considered intentionality as a basic property of our inner life. All our thoughts, perceptions, and feelings are connected to objects; more specifically, they are about or directed to those objects. We *think*, for example, of the *ballet* we saw last night. We *dream* of eating a *banana split*. We *watch* the *sun* set, *fear* a *terrorist act*, *smell* the aroma of *coffee*. All these activities are clearly linked with objects, and this linkage is critical to our understanding of them. Unlinking them renders the activities senseless. Can we fear without fearing something? What would fearing without an object even mean?

Pain, however, defies this property. Unlike other inner experiences, it doesn't take an object. Think of a bad headache, a convulsing menstrual cramp, or a shooting pain down the leg. What are these experiences about? What object inside or outside of us are they directed toward? Nothing readily comes to mind. This is why pain, according to Emily Dickinson, draws a "Blank," or turns back on itself—the only thing pain is about is itself. The consequences of this lack of intentionality, as Dickinson and Styron attest, are devastating; the absence of objects translates into an absence of the concreteness and palpability that objects lend to inner experience. Pain remains unmoored and elusive, "unimaginable" and "indescribable."

What is there to see or talk about when the *what* takes on the quality of blankness or darkness?

As the phenomenologists recognized, intentionality is critical to inner experience because it provides a structure and significance it otherwise would not possess. We don't love aimlessly; we love *this man* or *that woman* or *this dog*—objects that make our loving (and thinking and fearing) meaningful. In addition, intentionality allows inner experience to be exteriorized, to be expressed in language. Thinking and fearing are tied not just to *any* objects but specifically to objects that exist in a space that is accessible to others. When we attempt to communicate these personal and subjective experiences, we cannot do so without pointing to these "outer" objects. Certainly the love I feel for my wife may be difficult to convey, just as the aroma of coffee might be. But at least my feelings are anchored in a world that other people have the potential to move around in. Friends can meet my wife. They can see the coffee brewing and smell it for themselves. The object of the inner experience, we might say, "objectifies" that experience; it gives us something to point at and talk about. Other people will never feel exactly as I do about my wife or the aroma of coffee, but they can approach my feelings through a familiar world of shared objects.

Not so with pain. Remember how effective William Styron was at recreating the setting and details that preceded his breakdown. He eloquently writes about the signs, streets, and hotel he stayed in, conveying a vivid sense of what Paris was like and how he felt on the eve of his depression. But when the pain strikes and he tries to communicate it, he has nothing to grab on to. Unmoored, the pain is everywhere and nowhere. This absence, as Freud recognized over a century ago, is perhaps *the* defining characteristic of all kinds of pain, whether the psychological pain of depression and mourning or the physical pain of an open wound:

> Yet it cannot be for nothing that the common usage of speech
> should have created the notion of internal, mental pain and have

treated the feeling of loss of object [the loss of a loved one, for example, in the case of grief] as equivalent to physical pain.

The complex of melancholia behaves like an open wound, drawing to itself cathectic energies . . . from all directions and emptying the ego until it is totally impoverished.

Pain, then, by not being connected to *objects*, is amorphous. And by not being connected to *objects in the shared world*, it resists meaning and language. Finally, this lack of intentionality reaches beyond language and affects our experience of life as a whole. It substantiates the "ferocious inwardness" (Styron) we feel in pain. By not relating to anything outside of us, pain shatters our sense of being as a being-in-the-world and isolates us from others. The wall envisioned by the characters in Hemingway's and Solzhenitsyn's stories is not just in our minds—it is real.

A POSSIBLE EXCEPTION

Pain isn't always unconnected to the outside world. Unlike our previous examples of depression, headache, and lower back pain, there are occasions when pain seems more external. George S, for example, when he was wheeled into the emergency room after his accident, had multiple bruises and bleeding wounds, some with broken bone fragments protruding from them. So did the two other emergencies that morning: a woman who suffered severe burns to the left side of her body and a man who was shot six times in the neck and chest.

Surely in these instances, when pain is associated with damage to the surface of the body, things are not so indeterminate for the sufferer. Here *there are objects* linked to the pain—the visible injuries to the body (the gaping wounds and blistering skin) along with their causal agents (the careening car, the boiling water, and the automatic gun). And these objects, unlike the invisible goings-on that take place inside the body in the case of a headache, *are accessible* to others. So at least in these instances, the pain shouldn't seem entirely private, should be easier to communicate, and should be more difficult for a reasonable person to dismiss.

All this is true, and we will return to these scenarios later on, for they provide the raw material that can be used to create a language of pain in the far more common instances where no objects are present. For now, however, we must recognize that the presence of wounds and guns doesn't actually connect pain to the external world in the same way that objects of other inner experiences do. As we discussed, the property of intentionality suggests that inner experiences are *inseparable* from objects; thinking is a meaningful activity only if we are thinking of *something*. The relationship between experience and object is a necessary one.

Although we have been conditioned by personal experience and a long tradition in science to equate pain with injury (or objects that cause injury), they are not actually equatable. The relationship between experience and object in this case is much more arbitrary. We can easily think of instances where there is mild pain or even no pain at all despite serious injuries. Most famously, the physician Dr. Henry Beecher, reporting from the battlefields of World War II, observed that "three-quarters of badly wounded men, although they have received no morphine for hours, have so little pain that they do not want pain relief medication. . . . This is a puzzling thing." And the converse is equally true. We can easily think of instances when there is little trauma and damage to the body and yet a person complains of excruciating pain—in fibromyalgia, migraine, and a host of other chronic pain syndromes.

Observations like these and the basic scientific research they have spawned paved the way for a radical revision in our understanding of pain. Pain is no longer thought of as a signal that goes from a damaged area of the body directly to the brain. Instead, the signal can be influenced at various points along the way and can even be sounded in the absence of damage altogether. The scientific basis for what

Ronald Melzack, a pioneer in the field, called the "variable connection" between pain and injury is that our brains don't simply experience pain but must actively perceive it. Moreover, the perception varies among different people because of many factors beyond the presence or extent of injury: the size and activity of certain areas in an individual's brain, specific genes that determine pain thresholds, and one's emotional and cognitive state at the time of injury (people who are distracted tend to experience less pain, for example, and people who are anxious experience more pain).

The fact that we can separate pain from the only relatively consistent external object that accompanies it (injury) undermines its connection to the outside world and inevitably shifts the experience to the private realm again. So even when a visible injury (or the gun that caused the injury) is present, the pain still appears to be more *inside* us than *outside* us. Weeks later, when the gun is gone and the wound has healed, there still may be pain. This kind of disconnection never happens with other inner experiences and explains why a sufferer feels detached from the world—and why observers of pain, even doctors, can remain skeptical about someone else's pain.

THE INACCESSIBILITY OF THE BODY

The second reason for the elusiveness of pain involves the indeterminacy of bodily experience in general. In the last chapter, the issue of inaccessibility was raised in the context of observing pain. Since observers can never experience the pain of another person, they can never truly grasp or validate those experiences. But here, inaccessibility also becomes an issue for the sufferers themselves. Pain thrusts us into a world that—however intimate and familiar since it is the world of our own bodies—remains fundamentally opaque.

This may sound strange considering the dramatic change over the past few decades in our understanding of the body and its far-reaching influence. No longer do most people subscribe to the tradition (rightly or wrongly attributed to Descartes) that views the body as an inferior entity, distinct from the primary thinking mind, or *cogito*. Nowadays, we speak of being embodied, meaning that mind and body are inextricably linked and on equal planes. Moreover, this commitment to embodiment has pervasive influences on all facets of life, from the way we think and speak to the way we define ourselves and make moral decisions. The body, we have come to realize, directs us just as much as we direct it. All of these facts would indicate that we are very much aware of the body at all times, even when engaged in activities that seemingly have nothing to do with it, like language, thought, politics, and ethics.

We could also say that our awareness of the body in general exists at the individual level. Physicians like me are often humbled by the uncanny sense that some patients have about what goes on inside their bodies. Deciding that something is wrong with them, or, less commonly, that nothing is wrong, patients will blatantly contradict the assessment of their doctors and the "objective" data gleaned from sophisticated medical tests. Often they turn out to be right. On a certain level, they know their bodies better than outsiders, even professionals. I am reminded of a patient of mine with intractable pruritus (itching) that seemed to have no cause; bloodwork, skin biopsies, and a CAT scan were all negative. But the patient, a young dentist, was not satisfied. Like Hemingway's Harry, he knew that something was wrong and so pushed for another series of tests three months after the first. Sure enough, he was right. The second CAT scan showed slightly enlarged lymph nodes, and a few weeks later my patient received the first round of chemotherapy for Hodgkin's lymphoma.

How then should we characterize our relationship to the body? Are we always aware of and knowledgeable about it, or is it more of a black box to us? The truth lies somewhere in the middle. On the one hand, our bodies are literally with us all the time, and their presence, as contemporary thinkers have shown, cannot fail to influence us. On the other hand, this ongoing presence doesn't translate into transparency. Our knowledge of our bodies is limited. We know them on a more instinctive, almost primitive or "gut" level, which is why we have difficulty explaining or talking about them. This kind of practical knowledge is involved in activities like learning how to ride a bicycle: we don't have to think about it, we just do it. In a similar way, we don't have to think about our body, we use and live it. My patient's conviction that something was wrong with him was intuitive. It didn't come from deductive reasoning, and he couldn't easily convey it to his doctor or wife. But as sure as he was about the knowledge, its resistance to representation led him to search determinedly for confirmation in the objective world.

We can't know the body in a more thoughtful and expressive way because two fundamental modes of acquiring knowledge are lacking: perceptual access and the judgment of others. If someone gives us a strange object, for example, and asks us to familiarize ourselves with it, we will initially examine the object with our senses. We'll look at it, touch and listen to it, maybe even smell and taste it. After we form an impression, we'll ask other people for theirs. We might go a step further by referring to a textbook or encyclopedia. And if we want to be more scientific still, we can measure the object with standard measuring devices—a ruler, thermometer, spectrometer.

But these avenues of knowledge are problematic when it comes to the experience of the body. First, the major sensory organs, designed to illuminate the outside world, provide us with a very partial picture. We can see and touch only some of the body's surface and can smell and listen to only a fraction of its interior. Second, the minor sensory organs involved in monitoring the inside of the body—for example, pain and itch receptors—provide us with information that pales in comparison to what we receive from the external world. They may tell us that *something* is happening *somewhere* in the body, but they typically can be no more specific about the event or the location. On occasion, those organs are not merely vague but downright deceptive. In the case of referred pain, for example, we might feel pain in our arm even though it actually originates in the heart. With phantom pain, we feel it in a limb that is gone.

In addition to providing meager information, these internal sensory organs, unlike the major sensory organs, are beyond our control and cannot be fine-tuned. If we need to see better, we might squint or shield our eyes with a hand. If we need to discriminate between different sounds, we can muffle our ears. We can't, however, magnify or hone in on our internal sensations. Last, there is no way to enhance our impressions by asking for outside help. It's true that we might consult textbooks and doctors about what is happening inside our body, but they cannot share or verify our experience of such internal happenings. No wonder it is so important for patients to describe their sensations in as much detail as possible, for only they are privy to such information, and only they can make it available for doctors to interpret.

Pain continually eludes our grasp and frustrates us with its elusiveness. We·feel the need to pin it down and understand it better. This need is an integral part of pain and yet another feature that distinguishes it from other inner experiences. The aroma of coffee (which is associated with an external object), for example, or a mild itch (which is not) may seem at times just as difficult to conceptualize and express. But these difficulties don't typically distress us as pain does. Pain possesses an urgency the other cases lack—an urgency that can rise to the level of life-and-death. It *demands* a response, both a physical one, like withdrawing one's hand from a flame, and an intellectual one, like needing to find out where the hurt is coming from and, more important, *why it is happening*. The sociologist David Bakan writes that attempting to understand pain is already responding to the imperative of pain itself:

No experience demands and insists upon interpretation in the same way. Pain forces the question of its meaning, and especially of its cause, insofar as cause is an important part of its meaning. In those instances in which pain is intense and intractable and in which its causes are obscure, its demand for an interpretation is most naked, manifested in the sufferer asking, "Why?"

The demand for interpretation is a demand for knowledge, but not the intuitive, inarticulate kind we normally associate with the body. We want to know pain in the way we know the external world. We want this in the hope that it can convert the opacity of the body into a transparency, allowing us to see into our pain and deal with it more effectively.

THE CRISIS OF PAIN

When our instinctive attitude to pain is combined with pain's elusiveness, the experience rises to the level of crisis. The quintessential private experience, pain severs our engagement with the world and thrusts us inward. Our isolation is exacerbated by the incomprehension of others. Naturally, we try to communicate our feelings, but the language runs dry. It does so because in confronting the experience, in trying to make sense of what is happening, we see only darkness. Both the lack of intentionality and the difficulties in knowing the body corroborate the darkness and the inexpressibility of the experience. It becomes a vicious cycle. In pain we are alone.

3

The Public Side of Pain

> A *picture* held us captive. And we could not get
> outside it, for it lay in our language and language
> seemed to repeat it inexorably.
>
> —LUDWIG WITTGENSTEIN,
> *Philosophical Investigations*

In unraveling the reasons for pain's inexpressibility, we have painted an extremely bleak picture for the sufferer, bringing us directly back to Edward Munch's painting of the silent scream. The cards seem stacked against a person in pain, the obstacles insurmountable. One begins to feel the sense of futility that those in pain often feel: Why bother making an attempt to speak?

All this is quite true—unless, of course, the picture we have been painting is not entirely accurate, unless the obstacles confronting the sufferer are not as daunting as they appear. By drawing on the work of the German philosopher Ludwig Wittgenstein, we will see that the wall separating the sufferer from others is more porous than we imagine; that we can actually share (to some degree) experiences like pain that we believe are private; and that however counterintuitive it seems, this shared or public side of pain is infinitely more meaningful than any strictly unsharable and private one. Emphasizing the public side of pain can change the mindset of sufferers so that that they no longer feel the futility of trying to breach the wall, no longer resign themselves to dwell in pain alone.

One of the giants of twentieth-century philosophy, Wittgenstein was initially known for his work in formal logic. Later in his career, though, he developed an interest in ordinary language. One of the chief claims of his book *Philosophical Investigations* is that observing language and the way it is used in everyday life can tell us a lot about our world and how things in the world acquire meaning. If we are good observers, we'll find that we're often very confused about how this occurs. A specific example is our belief that each of us has a richly meaningful private world. A part of that world, perhaps, can be communicated and shared with others, through language, gestures, pictures, and other avenues of expression. But that part, we believe, is negligible. No one else can experience the far larger part of our inner world—our deepest thoughts, feelings, and perceptions. And this part, the unsharable and incommunicable part, is clearly what is most important and what distinguishes us as individuals.

According to Wittgenstein, this picture is completely wrong and completely at odds with reality. It has to be, or else we wouldn't have functioning languages and mutual understanding. Just think about it. If every person were responsible for assigning his or her own meanings to words, there is more than a good chance that we would all end up with different meanings. If that were the case, how on earth could we ever live together in communities and understand each other? The situation would resemble the chaos of the biblical city of Babel. Yet clearly it does not. Therefore, argues Wittgenstein, we had better change the way we think about our private worlds.

It shouldn't be surprising that Wittgenstein chooses pain to make his case. If you want to deflate the significance of the private sphere, you might as well confront its most distinguished resident. If Wittgenstein could show that even pain is not as private as we believe, then surely the entire house of cards would come crashing down.

Wittgenstein's arguments are relatively straightforward. All we have to do, he tells us, is to keep an open mind and observe how language is used, not by professional philosophers but by ordinary people. When we do so, we'll find, despite all our bellyaching about the inadequacy of language, *that we have a word for pain*, which is, of course, "pain." Not only do we have a word, we have a functional word, one that we use all the time and that other people understand. When a man grabs his chest and says he feels a tightening pain, an observer will sympathize and call for help. If a jogger happens to trip in front of me and says she's in so much pain she can't stand up, I won't turn and walk the other way; I'll kneel down and offer my hand. "Just try in a real case," Wittgenstein challenges us, "to doubt someone else's fear or pain."

That is not say that there aren't situations when suffering is overlooked, when the utterance "I am in pain" is questioned. It happens, as we saw earlier, even in medicine, a calling specifically dedicated to the alleviation of suffering. But we mustn't overemphasize those situations. For the most part, reasonable people will respond in appropriate ways to someone claiming to be in pain.

Despite our instinctive beliefs about inner experience, we have a working language of pain. If we acknowledge that we do, argues Wittgenstein, we must also accept its implication: namely, that we can't keep talking about the absolute privacy of pain. A working language—one in which words are uttered, received, and acted on—implies some degree of mutual understanding. When the injured jogger tells me she is in so much pain she can't walk, I am sympathetic and try to help. My feelings and subsequent response indicate that the woman's experience has been communicated. Therefore her experience *isn't* completely private. Her pain is accessible to me. It is, to an extent, made public.

Now, this is as simple as an argument gets, one that is exceedingly difficult to disprove. But the skeptic in us, like the interlocutor in Wittgenstein's *Investigations* and the fictional and real-life sufferers we encountered earlier, will probably not be satisfied. Fine, they may reluctantly agree, pain is universal to a degree, part of the human condition as it were, and therefore sharable in a sense, but only in the *most limited and superficial sense.* There's got to be a lot more to it than that. What pain feels like to me, no one else can possibly know and no one else can possibly share. It's inside me. Private. Mine and mine alone. That's the most important part of the experience—*the essence of my pain.*

We can call this response a compromise solution: the two-language, two-meaning compromise. There may be a public word and meaning for pain, but there is also a private word and a private meaning. And we can't help but believe that the latter—the private and unsharable part of pain—is what's most important about the experience.

But this too is completely wrong. The only part of pain that is truly private is having the experience: I have it, you don't, and you can never have it in the same way I do. But as soon as language and meaning enter the picture, we have moved beyond the private experience and into the public realm of sharing it. Language and meaning are incompatible with private experience. They can never rely on personal, subjective criteria.

Wittgenstein presents a more formal argument, which has been called the private-language argument, to show why this must be so. It takes the form of a *reductio ad absurdum*, an argument that works to demonstrate that a certain premise leads to untenable and absurd consequences. Briefly, if pain (the word and its meaning) refers to a private experience, then

1. **How could we ever teach the concept of pain to another person?** We couldn't, for it would be impossible to impart something private to another person and equally impossible for the other person to learn it. But we can and indeed do teach our children what pain means, and they subsequently demonstrate their understanding of it. So, then, how can we maintain that pain—the word, the concept, the meaning we ascribe to it— refers to a solely private, individual experience?

2. **How would we ever know that another person was in pain?** We couldn't. It would only be known to one person, unless we were able to enter that person's consciousness. Yet for the most part we do know when other people are in pain: We feel terrible for the person with a blinding headache, we rush the accident victim to the hospital—which again disproves the absolute privacy of pain.

3. **How can we be sure that we use the concept correctly and consistently?** In order to achieve consistency and accuracy in language, we depend on other people. If we're not sure about a word or concept, we ask another person for his judgment or we refer to some standardized set of rules or reference guide. But we certainly couldn't do that if pain were private, since how could private criteria be publicized or standardized? In fact, a private language probably wouldn't even work for the individual, for a Robinson Crusoe stuck on an uninhabited island. In the absence of any objective criteria, how would Crusoe be sure that what he called pain one day was the same sensation he experienced the following day? If all he had to rely on was his own memory, it would be impossible to guarantee any consistency.

And even if we disregard these reservations, even if we grant the possibility of a person's creating his own language in isolation, Wittgenstein raises a final rhetorical question:

4. **What would be the purpose of a language based on private experience?** If we really think about it, the notion of private languages and private meanings is absurd, completely devoid of any practical benefits. Why would I need to tell myself something I already know? It would be no different than presenting oneself with a gift:

> Why can't my right hand give my left hand money?—My right hand can put it into my left hand. My right hand can write a

deed of gift and my left hand a receipt. But the further practical consequences would not be those of a gift. When the left hand has taken the money from the right, we shall ask: "Well, and what of it?"

Language, we come to realize, is a practice that involves many people and that must be anchored in a public, shared space where it can be agreed upon, negotiated, and renegotiated over time. Otherwise it would be useless.

So if we exclude language and meaning from our inner worlds, what is left? What remains of that supposedly substantial private sphere we stubbornly cling to? Very little indeed, and this is precisely Wittgenstein's great insight. Our notion of living in two separate worlds, the private one that we alone know (major) and the public one that we share with others (minor), is wildly exaggerated. In fact, the private world is an illusion, a sham. It consists for the most part in having experiences—feeling pain, seeing colors, falling in love. And while these experiences are quite real and private in the sense that they are had by only a single person—although many people feel pain, see color, and fall in love—they are very much like our experience of the body: exceedingly vague and amorphous.

They are also very much like the book on the language of pain that was in my head before I was able to write it down on paper or talk about it coherently with another person—in short, not a book at all, but a chaotic sea of undeveloped ideas. Still, I'd like to say that I had some good ideas, preliminary as they were at one point. Rubbish, Wittgenstein would counter. Let's be honest with ourselves. At that preliminary point, there was nothing in my head, nor did I possess anything substantive:

In what sense have you *got* what you are talking about and saying only you have got it? Do you possess it? You do not even *see* it. Must you not really say that no one has got it? And this too is clear: if as a matter of logic you exclude other people's having something, it loses its sense to say that you have it.

Only by giving our inchoate ideas and experiences form—by assigning them words and meanings, through language, gestures, or whatever other form of expression we choose—do we transcend the profoundly limited world of the self and move into the only world that can have meaning and language, the shared, public one. Wittgenstein would surely have agreed with Maurice Merleau-Ponty's concept of being-in-the-world: "Man is in the world and only in the world does he know himself."

If we agree with Wittgenstein, we must acknowledge that part of the difficulty we have in expressing pain is in our minds. Regardless of whether we blame culture, tradition, or poor old Descartes, we can't help but prioritize and cling to our private worlds. All we see in pain is isolation, the wall that separates us from others. But why not make room for the possibility that we can breach the wall, that we can share our experience? Why not acknowledge that we actually *do* breach that wall and do so on a regular basis? We have a word for pain, a functioning word, and that fact makes the experience *sharable* to an extent. This is not to minimize the feelings of those in pain. The shift of perspective, the turning inward, the sense of isolation—these are all very real. Moreover, there are still formidable obstacles that prevent us from being able to express pain: its lack of intentionality and the inaccessibility of the body. My point is simply that we mustn't focus exclusively on the dividing wall that pain erects, but work to remove as many bricks as possible so that we might see through to the other side. We must break with the illusions of the private world and focus instead on the public and sharable one.

I also don't mean to suggest that the generic word "pain" captures the experience of pain in full. There is no doubt that when we use the word, what we share of our experience is quite limited and hardly satisfying for the sufferer. But the fact that we have a word, the fact that language can make inroads into what we consider our most intimate and private sphere, should give us hope that we might be able to communicate even better. Wittgenstein's work provides an opening in the formidable wall of pain. In subsequent chapters, we will seize on this opening and try to enlarge it as much as possible by searching for ways to convey the feelings and nuances that make up the experience of pain.

4

Man's Puny Inexhaustible Voice

When the last dingdong of doom has clanged and
faded from the last worthless rock hanging tideless
in the last red and dying evening, that even then
there will still be one more sound: that of [man's]
puny inexhaustible voice, still talking.

—WILLIAM FAULKNER,
Nobel Prize acceptance speech, 1950

Wittgenstein urges us to modify our instinctive belief that
pain is unsharable. As long as we can generate a working language for pain, then it has to be sharable. We may not be satisfied
with the extent of its sharability, but that shouldn't direct us back
into our private world for a more meaningful description. As both
philosophers (Wittgenstein and Merleau-Ponty) and sufferers (William Styron and George S) point out, we will find nothing there
except darkness.

But perhaps deep down we know this on some level; we know that
our beliefs aren't entirely accurate and may even be self-destructive.
Certainly there are plenty of times when we don't go silently into the
night—times, especially when the pain is not at its worst, when we
do try as hard as we can to breach the wall. Although Styron tells us
that he could only balk and stutter when the pain struck, he doesn't
remain mute (or "wall-eyed," as he says) for long. As soon as the pain
subsides, he begins to speak again. Eventually he writes a book about

his pain, sharing his experience with others eloquently, even the balking and stuttering part of it.

Despite the overwhelming pull inward, there is always a pull in the opposite direction. We rarely withdraw without a fight. Like Faulkner's apocalyptic survivor, most of us will struggle to overcome the wall by ex-pressing our pain (literally, pushing it outward) and attempting to share it with others.

If we listen carefully, we can hear this commitment in Wittgenstein's dialogue with his imaginary interlocutor in the *Philosophical Investigations*. Despite the many arguments Wittgenstein showers on him, the interlocutor refuses to believe that the essence and meaning of his pain don't lie inside him. *This*, insists the interlocutor stubbornly, pointing to the sensation, *is the important thing*. But we mustn't miss the contradiction in his behavior. Although the interlocutor is literally pointing in one direction (to the inner world), he is at the same time figuratively pointing in the opposite direction (to the outer one) by continuing to talk. He wants Wittgenstein to understand how he feels—he is desperate to transcend the isolating boundaries of his private world.

The scene demonstrates a blatant inconsistency in our behavior when it comes to pain. We cling to the interiority of the experience and subvert it at the same time. We see this with Styron, who tells us that pain is "inexpressible" in a full-length book on the subject. Virginia Woolf, too, felt increasingly isolated in illness and decided that the experience "cannot be imparted." Yet in the act of writing "On Being Ill," she invites us into her sickbed—under the covers, so to speak—and articulately *imparts* her feelings. Likewise, Emily Dickinson equates pain with blankness but does so in a poem that is anything but blankness. And Edvard Munch gives us an eloquent representation of pain in a sufferer whose scream cannot be heard. So while these artists claim that suffering is a solitary and inexpressible experience, their works contradict that message; they are sharing their experience with those who view their paintings and read their words, even as they recognize that the experience can't be communicated in full.

George S, the chronic pain patient who becomes depressed, also doesn't shut himself off completely. He still drags himself to doctors for scheduled appointments and manages on occasion to express his feelings, sometimes with words but mostly with gestures. He becomes more talkative with a patient he recently met in an Internet chat room. The man had an almost identical experience after a failed surgery to correct a ruptured disk. Not only can he sympathize with George's frustration, but he may also be able to help. A new orthopedic procedure, he e-mails George, is being tested at some of the bigger academic hospitals. George should look into it. For the first time in what seems like an eternity, George feels hopeful.

It is practically impossible to extinguish our need to remain engaged with the world. It is as instinctive as, and perhaps insepa-rable from, the will to survive. The renowned psychiatrist and con-centration camp survivor Viktor Frankl recognized and wrote about this basic need after his release from Auschwitz. Even in the most extreme instances of suffering, we yearn to move beyond the bound-aries of self and find some semblance of meaning. Even in instances when the question "Why?" confronts us most intensely—*Why is this nightmare happening to me? Why not just kill myself and end the pain?*—the majority of people don't submit to the inward spiral. They manage to move forward and outward: in a joke shared between inmates, as Frankl suggests in *Man's Search for Meaning*; or in the hope that one might be reunited with a spouse or a child; or, in Frankl's own case, the desire to finish and publish the book he had been writing before he was captured.

All kinds of suffering, whether it arises from natural causes (ill-ness) or man-made ones (the Holocaust), isolate us. But as detached from the world as we feel, most of us will do whatever we can to find our way back. Our survival depends on it.

Joan Didion once wrote that she tells stories "in order to live." But perhaps it was not until recently that the full measure of that astonishing claim was brought home to her. On December 30, 2003, her husband and best friend of over forty years died. She was racked with a grief that reminds us of Emily Dickinson's blankness:

> Nor can we know ahead of the fact (and here lies the difference between grief as we imagine it and grief as it is) the unending absence that follows, the void, the very opposite of meaning, the relentless succession of moments during which we will confront the experience of meaningless itself.

Nine months and five days later, nothing had changed, and yet that day marked the beginning of her escape from the void, for it was then that she took up her pen to write about her experience in what would eventually materialize into a book, *The Year of Magical Thinking*. She replaces the absence with presence, a presence that will bear meaning both for herself and for others. Through writing Didion obliterates solitude and invites others (for writing implies an audience of readers) to share her grief.

The same urge to transcend the self and establish community is responsible for one of the most famous passages in all of English literature. In 1663, following the death of his wife and five children, John Donne was stricken with relapsing fever, a life-threatening illness endemic in London at the time, which confined him to his bed, where he suffered for weeks without respite. Doctors and specialists were consulted. They tried everything from purges to leeches. But when he didn't respond, they gave up on Donne. Left for dead, terrified and alone, he experienced only one interruption of his solitude: the sporadic sound of church bells in the distance, indicating yet another death from the epidemic. Suddenly Donne realized that even then, in the midst of this awful predicament, he was not alone:

> No man is an island, entire of itself; every man is a piece of the continent, a part of the main. If a clod be washed away by the sea, Europe is the less, as well as if a promontory were, as well as if a

manor of thy friend's or of thy own were: any man's death diminishes me, because I am involved in mankind, and therefore never send to know for whom the bell tolls; it tolls for thee.

A more recent instance of what Faulkner dubbed the inexhaustibility of the human voice can be found in the extraordinary achievement of Jean-Dominique Bauby. At age forty-three, Bauby, the editor of French *Elle*, suffered a massive stroke that left him with what is known as "locked-in syndrome." Completely and permanently paralyzed, he didn't shrivel up and submit. When he figured out that he could still blink one eye, he managed (with the help of a speech therapist) to create an alphabet based on the number of blinks. He taught others his alphabet and thereby communicated with them. He ultimately wrote a book about his ordeal, *The Diving Bell and the Butterfly*, though, sadly, he died a few days after it was published. Of course, Bauby's desire to communicate had a practical side—he wanted to be able to tell his nurses and doctors of his pain, hunger, and other needs. But at the same time, there was much more to it. Finding language was liberating for Bauby. It freed him from the imprisonment of his sick body, allowing the butterfly of his imagination to escape. Bauby was no longer alone.

We too can relieve the solitude of pain by reaching out to family and friends, by talking to other patients in the clinic or in Internet chat rooms, by communicating through gestures or drawings. The medium or level of mastery is less important than the process. One is reminded of Chekhov's short story "Heartache," about a lowly cabdriver who has just lost his son. All he wants is to talk to someone, anyone, even his abusive passengers, who laugh and curse at him. He "thirsts for speech" and the companionship it brings. But no one will listen. Just when it appears that he will carry his grief to bed, he finds a willing listener at last: his horse. And despite the pathos of the driver's situation, we as readers can't help but feel that even this one-sided conversation will have a good effect, that to some degree it will lessen the poor man's pain.

As we move to the next part of this book—generating a language for pain despite the formidable obstacles in our path—we should bear in mind the insights of thinkers and sufferers discussed in the past two chapters. First, Wittgenstein assures us that we *can* communicate what we hold to be most private, but to do so, we must rely on the public and sharable aspects of those experiences. And second, courageous sufferers like Frankl and Bauby assure us that no matter how extreme the ordeal, it's almost impossible to extinguish the desire to break down the pain wall. Inexhaustible, our voice, no matter how puny it may seem to us, will continue to sound as long as we live.

PART II

THE
SOLUTION

Metaphor and Worldmaking

> Our ordinary ways of imparting information about
> our own sensations consist in making certain sorts
> of references to what we think could be established
> in anyone's observations of common objects. We
> describe what is personal to ourselves in neutral or
> impersonal terms. Indeed, our descriptions would
> convey nothing unless couched in such terms.
>
> —GILBERT RYLE, *The Concept of Mind*

Stephen Dedalus is sent to a Jesuit boarding school in Ireland as a child. It is his first time away from home. He is shy and lonely. The other boys in his class have formed cliques, and Stephen is left out and teased. One day Wells, the class bully, pushes him into a muddy ditch, and soon after Stephen catches a cold. His classmates and teachers recognize the changes in Stephen's body; at times his face is red and at other times pale. They ask if he is sick, but Stephen doesn't know how to reply. He senses something is wrong but hasn't yet acquired the vocabulary of illness. He can't match his feelings with words that he could pass on to his classmates and teachers, thereby exacerbating his isolation.

But Stephen is no ordinary child. James Joyce's alter ego in *A Portrait of the Artist as a Young Man*, he possesses a vivid imagination and a precocious way with language. To make sense of his illness, he radically reinvents his world by drawing on familiar objects. He imagines a sink within his body that alternately runs with hot and cold water:

The white look of the lavatory made him feel cold and then hot. There were two cocks that you turned and water came out: cold and hot. He felt cold and then a little hot: and he could see the names printed on the cocks. That was a very queer thing.

Eventually the infection spreads to Stephen's ears. Again, he doesn't know that the pain he experiences is called an earache. Instead he remembers the time he rode a train at night:

He leaned his elbows on the table and shut and opened the flaps of his ears. Then he heard the noise of the refectory every time he opened the flaps of his ears. It made a roar like a train at night. And when he closed the flaps the roar was shut off like a train going into a tunnel. That night at Dalkey the train had roared like that and then, when it went into the tunnel, the roar stopped. He closed his eyes and the train went on, roaring and then stopping: roaring again, stopping.

The pain becomes the roar and stop of the train, just as the fever and chills are transformed into the hot and cold running water of the sink. Young Stephen, despite the obstacles, manages to communicate his private experiences and does so much more effectively than he could have accomplished with conventional words.

Stephen's situation closely approximates the crisis of pain. More important, it provides a resolution to the crisis through metaphor. By talking of what we don't understand in terms of what we do understand, metaphor gives us words and objects where there were none, clarity where there was murkiness, and the potential to share where there was loneliness.

THE CRISIS

Illness reminds us that we are separate from other people—that we are discrete entities bounded by our bodies and that we have experiences that others cannot have. It's not that we are unaware of these issues when healthy and pain-free. But illness reminds us of them with an intensity and urgency that is not present in other situations. Though it may be upsetting that my wife, Daniella, doesn't see the incredible sunsets at Fire Island the same way I do, I can live with that, just as I can live with the fact that I can't precisely convey to her how the aroma of coffee in the morning smells to me. As intimate as we are, my wife and I are two different people who can share only so much.

But such calm rationalization doesn't work when it comes to illness and in particular pain. Here the issue of subjectivity and separateness seems acute and intolerable. On a practical level, we need other people to understand how we feel so that they can take care of us, so that they can bring us to doctors and administer medicine. But we also need other people on a more existential level. As William Styron shows in his memoir, the "aching solitude" that accompanies pain *hurts* just as much as, and in some cases more than, the pain itself. David Foster Wallace, another prominent writer and sufferer, would agree. "The depressed person," he writes:

> was in terrible and unceasing emotional pain, and the impossibility of sharing or articulating this pain was itself a component of the pain and a contributing factor in its essential horror.

We might say that illness and pain not only remind us of our separateness but urge us to do something about it, to escape by reaching beyond the self to the world of family and friends. The problem is that the escape route is blocked by a formidable obstacle: language eludes us. In Stephen's case, it's a matter of not having mastered language. But even when we're older and have richer vocabularies, the experiences still seem "indescribable" (Styron) and "unimpartable"(Woolf). The resistance to language in turn reinforces the solitude. Stephen's inability to understand and answer the question repeatedly posed to him—*Are you sick?*—makes him feel even more isolated. A vicious cycle develops. This is why we refer to illness and pain in particular as crisis situations.

THE SOLUTION

Despite the obstacles, Stephen finds a way to speak. He responds to the absence of illness by becoming a creator, by engaging in what the philosopher Nelson Goodman calls worldmaking. This kind of creation, however, is not like creation in the biblical sense, where something comes from nothing. The world for us mortals is what is given to us; its contents cannot be changed. But how we see the world *can* change and be manipulated, which is why worldmaking, according to Goodman, is more a recreating or a remaking. For Stephen the facts are as follows: *inside* him are sensations he doesn't understand and cannot speak about; *outside* are things he does understand and can speak about. And because this situation is intolerable, he needs to alter it. He does so by mixing up categories, by taking from the things he does understand in order to illuminate the things he does not. He does so, that is, by metaphor, one of the most powerful means of worldmaking at our disposal. Metaphor exchanges absence for presence, darkness for light, and silence for language.

Stephen's symptoms (fever, chills, earache) are as real as any of the objects in his environment, but they lack the palpability and structure of those objects. Nor are they directly linked with objects that can lend them some of their palpability and structure—as the love object might, for example, to the felt experience of love. This objectlessness or lack of intentionality becomes extremely frustrating for Stephen. Through metaphor, he borrows from the world of form and meaning and projects what he borrows onto his interior sensations. The bathroom sink is now situated in his body (though the metaphor works in the opposite direction too, with Stephen's sensations projected onto the bathroom sink). By connecting his symptoms with objects, he objectifies them—literally turns them into objects—conferring on them a presence they once lacked.

A second consequence of Stephen's worldmaking is a gain in knowledge. The body for us, especially its interior, is opaque. Our means of accessing and understanding it are limited. This stems, as we saw earlier, from perceptual limitations, the inherent indeterminacy of bodily sensation, and our inability to check with outside sources. For Stephen, all this translates into a lack of knowledge. Metaphor, however, allows him to improve the situation considerably. By connecting his symptoms (the lesser-known entities) to the sink and the train (the better-known ones), Stephen can now see and feel and touch the body's interior. Moreover, he can conceptualize and reason about what happens there. We might say that Stephen uses metaphor in much the same way a scientist might. Four hundred years ago, when William Harvey dispensed with the prevailing theories of his day and first envisioned the heart as a pump, he remade the entire field of human physiology. It's not that the heart *is* a pump or that an earache *is* the roar and stop of the train. The metaphors operate like models, or conceptual vehicles, that can be used to organize and further investigate the body and other phenomena. In this way, they contribute to our ever-evolving base of knowledge.

Finally, Stephen's act of worldmaking reverses the inward pull of illness. Before metaphor, Stephen's world had been reduced to his private and inexpressible experience of his body as it responded to infection. But unlike Wittgenstein's interlocutor, who tries (and inevitably fails) to communicate his pain by pointing inward, Stephen points in the opposite direction, outward to the sink and the roar of the train, objects that are situated in the shared, interpersonal world. By doing so, he makes what was initially a private experience a public one. Other people—in this case, the readers of

Joyce's novel—are now privy to what Stephen is feeling. Metaphor has enabled him to express his experience, in the etymological sense of pushing it outward (*expremere*). As a result, he has gained some control over it (by naming it) and is no longer alone, both of which help to relieve his pain.

METAPHOR AS DEVIATION OR NECESSITY

We found a solution to the crisis of pain in metaphor. Considering the context—a novel—this shouldn't be surprising. We expect to find rhetorical devices in literature. But is metaphor the only way to solve the crisis? Is there a more literal and direct way to do so, one that might be used by ordinary people in real situations, patients in clinics and hospitals, for example, who may not possess the rhetorical gifts of a James Joyce?

A visit to a pain clinic or an emergency room would suggest that there is not. When asked by a doctor to describe the pain in her leg, one patient responds that it is *burning*. A man with chronic emphysema says he feels like he is *being choked*. A young girl with abdominal discomfort speaks of *shooting* pains. A woman with pelvic pain believes something inside her is *tearing*. Other patients describe their pain as *pounding, stabbing, drilling, blinding, squeezing, wrenching, dragging*, and *grinding*.

The figurative nature of this language is immediately apparent. Patients who talk of stabbing or choking pain haven't actually been stabbed or choked. Nor have they been dragged, wrenched, or drilled on. Like Stephen Dedalus, they talk about their experience in terms of another experience, which, even if only imagined, is much more concrete and visible than their pain. In short, they enter the realm of rhetoric, specifically the realm of metaphor.

Naturally this raises many questions. If patients only imagine scenarios of stabbing and searing, how accurate and reliable are their reports? Does there even exist a less imaginary, more literal way to talk about pain? Then again, while the language of patients is blatantly metaphorical, how can we characterize it as such when it is used by ordinary people day in and day out? Isn't that how we define literal language, as opposed to the more literary kind that appears in novels and poetry?

The ubiquitous use of metaphor in the context of pain calls into question the very distinction between literal and metaphorical language. The language of pain *is* and *is not* metaphorical. On the one hand, it is indirect and patently false: it speaks of one subject in terms of another. On the other hand, everyone, from Joyce to the man in the street, seems to rely on it. There is no more literal or direct way to convey pain.

The problem with completely collapsing the distinction between metaphorical and literal language, however, is that the distinction seems crucial to understanding metaphor. Metaphor, after all, is a figure that "clothes" words with a presence that ordinary language lacks and a trope that involves a "turning" of ordinary language. Most theorists of metaphor, from Aristotle to Paul Ricoeur, emphasize this deviation—that is, the movement or transference from a home or familiar realm to an alien or unfamiliar realm. They do so because this characteristic allows us to recognize when we are in the midst of metaphor; the roaring of a train is clearly *not* the usual way we talk of earaches. Second, deviation helps explain how metaphor works. It provides the motivation for finding new meanings. Generating what the philosopher Donald Davidson calls a "bump on the head," deviation compels us to bring together two disparate entities to create a novel proximity. The roar and stop of the train is so different and original a way of talking about ear pain that it makes us stop and think about the similarities between the two entities. We may say that the more a metaphor deviates from ordinary language, the more suggestive and resonant it tends to be.

But what about metaphor and pain? How can we talk of deviation when there doesn't seem to be any literal language in the first place? If there's no literal language, then how can there be movement away from it? And if there's no movement, then how could there be a bump on the head that compels us to make new connections?

The truth is that the distinction between metaphor and literal language is incredibly slippery, not only in the context of pain but in all contexts. Once again pain, being the defining experience that it is, dramatically brings this fact to our attention. Many philosophers insist that there is no neutral rhetoric, that our so-called literal language is saturated with metaphor. But these metaphor-heavy accounts of language obscure the distinction between dead and living metaphor. Language is a dynamic activity. Novel metaphors create novel meanings (via deviation), but when used over and over again they lose their suggestivity (along with their deviation). Aging metaphors become an integral part of our literal language.

The words used by patients in the clinic are not as resonant as Joyce's language. They are, however, metaphorical. All share the motif of agency, which, as we will see in the next chapter, is the most common way we communicate pain. Stabbing, drilling, pounding all imply an agent or outside force (imagined and therefore metaphorical) that acts upon the body to cause pain. But because these words are used so frequently, they lack the suggestivity of truly vital metaphor; the bump on the head is a small one, if a bump at all.

Joyce's metaphors, in contrast, have a completely different feel. They generate a bump on the head that makes us *see and think and talk about* Stephen's illness in a radically new way. They behave like literary language in general. Ordinarily, the Russian formalists remind us, language is used so automatically that we become anesthetized to it. Only when poets stretch language in unfamiliar ways do we begin to *see* again—the words, that is, as well as what the words stand for.

FILLING VOIDS

By emphasizing deviation, philosophers have overlooked one of the most critical functions of metaphor. People in pain are not interested in reinvigorating the familiar by seeing it in terms of something unfamiliar; they don't create metaphor for effect. Their primary motivation is to fill a void, to find a way to make their pain real for themselves and others. In pain we don't choose metaphor but are forced in that direction because there is no literal language. It's either metaphor or continued absence.

For these reasons, a much better way of thinking about this particular class of metaphor is in terms of catachresis. Traditionally, catachresis was the rhetorical figure that provided names for things that have no names. According to Aristotle, because there is an asymmetry between language (which is finite) and the world (which is infinite), we will eventually run out of words and therefore need to economize, by extending the meaning of a particular word to cover additional objects. We refer, for example, to the "leg" of a table or the "foot" of a mountain.

These examples of catachresis are relatively banal instances of language extension. Like many simple substitution-type metaphors that operate at the level of single words, they lack the suggestivity and cognitive dimension of more complex metaphors. Contemporary philosophers' main criticism of traditional theory is its reliance on such simple substitutions, which cannot possibly account for the power of our best metaphors. The problem stems from a different understanding of language. Earlier theorists believed that language was a vehicle for our ideas, which have form and meaning to begin with and are then attached to words and thereby transmitted to other people. For them language has no influence on the way we think or the content of our thought (or at least their theories don't account for such influence).

Nowadays we have a higher regard for language. We recognize that language is inextricably entwined with our thoughts, which don't have form and meaning before they are put into words. Language is as much constitutive of our thoughts as it is illustrative of them. Nowhere is this more evident than in the realm of rhetoric. Metaphor in particular has the capacity to extend and even create new categories of thought.

In order to account for the change in our understanding of language and the potential of metaphor, contemporary philosophers have had to revise the older theories. Because they believe we think in terms of phrases and sentences as opposed to individual words, nominalism (of single words) had to be replaced with semantics (of word groupings and meanings). Contemporary philosophers speak of metaphor as an *interaction* between sentences, ideas, and categories rather than the *substitution* of words. Only in this way is it possible for metaphor to generate novel meanings and thoughts.

Unlike metaphor, however, catachresis was left untouched. This is unfortunate, because a change in the way we understand catachresis, identical to the change in the way we now understand metaphor, would explain a certain class of metaphor much better than theories of deviation and interaction. We can see this most clearly in the setting of pain. On the surface we are faced with a linguistic absence. But that is not to say we simply lack the means to transmit an experience that is already understood. As Wittgenstein makes clear, before language, the content of our inner experiences—the private, mysterious stuff inside what he calls the beetle box—is meaningless:

> The thing in the box has no place in the language game at all; not even as a *something*: for the box might even be empty. No, one can 'divide through' by the thing in the box; it cancels out, whatever it is.

What we truly lack in these instances is a way to *formulate* experience—to provide it with structure and form, thereby enabling us to think about and generate meanings for it.

And this is precisely what a contemporary vision of catachresis might be called upon to do. Not merely filling voids in our lexicon (providing names for the nameless), catachresis could be used to fill voids at much higher levels—semantic, conceptual, and epistemic. Moreover, filling these voids, *not* finding alternative ways of saying something, is the sole purpose of the exercise. While we need a second subject (the metaphorical vehicle) to do so, it is not the interaction between the two that should be emphasized. Metaphors of pain are first and foremost about pain (not about pain *and* the stabbing knife we connect it to). Finally, understanding metaphors of pain in terms of catachresis emphasizes their urgency and necessity. We don't voluntarily choose to speak metaphorically; we are forced into it.

In light of these considerations, we should modify our definition of pain. Pain threatens to destroy our language and conceptual abilities, leaving a void. The only way to represent that experience and fill the void is through metaphor:

Pain is an all-consuming interior experience that threatens to destroy everything except itself *and can only be described through metaphor*.

There are at least two other settings in which we rely on metaphor with similar urgency: religion and science. The primary object of religion, like pain, is characterized by absence. Although worshippers believe in the reality of God, that reality is beyond their grasp. By definition, God is remote and incomprehensible. How then can people talk about and understand God? Only indirectly and figuratively, as the twelfth-century Jewish scholar Maimonides noted apologetically in his *Guide for the Perplexed*. Believers speak of God as composed of matter, as possessing attributes, as existing in time, even though they know all this is false. They do so because, as Maimonides reminds us, the Torah can speak in only one language, the language of man. Metaphor is indispensable to religion, for without it there would be no way to approach God.

Metaphor is also critical in science, a discipline that strives for accuracy and simplicity and typically avoids literary language. Yet if science is ever to progress, if new and better theories of how the world works are ever to replace older ones, then we have to consider the existence of voids at the frontiers of knowledge, of phenomena that are at one point incompletely understood and that later on will become part of our collective knowledge. But how do scientists conceptualize (and communicate) what they don't yet fully understand, during those periods of scientific revolution that the historian Thomas Kuhn refers to as paradigm shifts? Faced with a similar kind of absence to that experienced by the sufferer of pain and the believer in God, scientists respond in the only way available to them. They fill the void by means of metaphor, by thinking of an inadequately or partially known subject in terms of a more fully known one, by mapping out the unknown subject onto the semantic points of the known.

In this way scientific metaphor is a conceptual vehicle that works to bridge gaps in knowledge. It allows us to think and speak about indeterminate phenomena without staking a claim to absolute truth—as when Harvey thought of the heart in terms of a pump; or when Maxwell thought of the electromagnetic field in terms of waves; or, most recently, when physicists began thinking of the elementary particles of matter in terms of oscillating strings (so-called string theory). It's not that physicists believe those particles *are* strings but that they believe they are *like* strings. There are similarities and differences between the two entities, nuances, and varying levels of complexity. Like any important scientific model, the metaphor is an approximation. It allows physicists to revise their description as time goes on, to inch closer and closer to the truth.

In fact, the truth value of catachretical metaphors may be irrelevant. Earlier we questioned the accuracy of pain reports recorded in the hospital and clinic. If patients have never been stabbed or shot, how accurate (and therefore trustworthy) can descriptions of pain as stabbing or shooting really be? And yet what would count as an entirely accurate and true description of pain? What would count as a true description of God? In any case where no direct or literal language is available to us, where we confront something that we cannot entirely know, where absolute truth is not a possibility, we have no choice but to rely on metaphor. Otherwise there would be only silence and darkness.

WORLDMAKING

There is perhaps no single unifying theory that can accommodate all kinds of metaphor. The most productive way of understanding metaphors of pain, though, is in terms of catachresis rather than interaction and deviation.

In the settings of pain, religion, and science, we are absolutely dependent on metaphor. It makes no sense in these instances to talk of metaphor as a figure (giving language more "bodily" presence) or as a trope (turning away from the literal to create dissonance). Nor does it make sense to talk of reinvigorating language and objects by seeing them in a fresh light. All these notions imply that we have a language that can represent the subject of metaphor *from the beginning*. They also imply that we have a choice in the matter, that we voluntarily mix categories and look forward to the unexpected results. But neither is the case. We don't have a way of understanding and talking about pain without metaphor. If we are to speak at all, we must use metaphor.

One cannot fail to be impressed by the power of metaphor. We reach for it in moments of extremity, at the margins and frontiers of our shared world—the very same moments, according to philosophers like Ernst Cassirer, Susanne Langer, and Richard Rorty, in which we depend on myth and symbol-making, activities that distinguish human beings from all other creatures. Catachretical metaphor allows us to break free and transcend the tethers of our solitary being and forge a community of shared language, beliefs, and knowledge. It is indeed world*making*.

An unfortunate part of life, pain offers us an extraordinary opportunity. It places us alongside the sufferer in these liminal situations, at the time before language is mastered (as in Stephen Dedalus's case) or at the frontiers of the knowable and expressible. It places us in the solitary space of what Maurice Merleau-Ponty calls primordial existence, a space of brute, anonymous being. By observing a sufferer fill that space through metaphor, we stand at the threshold where language and knowledge emerge from the void. We are, in essence, witnesses at their very birth.

6

The Weapon

I cannot conceptualize infinite pain without whips and scorpions, hot irons and other people.

—MICHAEL WALZER, *Just and Unjust Wars*

In the Kings County Hospital emergency room, a teenage boy is brought in by his mother. John clutches his belly and winces.

Where does it hurt? asks the doctor, leading them into an open examining room.

Here, the boy says, pointing to the lower right side of his abdomen. *But yesterday it was closer to my belly button.*

Does it hurt all the time or just some of the time?

Some of the time. It comes and goes. But it's coming a lot more now.

Does it feel like a dull aching sensation, or is it more sharp and piercing?

Like a knife, says John, *that's stabbing me in the belly.* He is wincing again and tightening his abdomen, as if he's trying to steel it against the next onslaught of the imaginary knife.

Despite his fear and discomfort, John has given a good description of his pain. The physical examination will no doubt confirm the doctor's initial impression. The boy will need emergency surgery to remove his ruptured appendix.

Rachel J's pain is different. For one thing, it's not as new and scary. A middle-aged nurse, Rachel has lived with migraines for as long as she can remember. In a strange way, the pain is like an old friend. That's why she doesn't rush to the ER but has a scheduled appointment at a pain clinic—a recent development in medicine, spurred on by the growing number of patients with chronic pain syndromes and the inability of general practitioners to help them. But as familiar as she is with her old friend, their encounters never get any easier. Each one is as bad as the preceding one, and after all this time, they have taken a toll.

For all these differences, Rachel uses the same kind of metaphor as the boy with appendicitis to describe her pain. "My migraines," she tells her doctor, "are not like other headaches. The pounding kind, for example, that feels like a hammer is coming down on your skull. Or when my sinuses act up and my head feels like it's being squeezed in a vise. The migraines are in a class by themselves. The pain is explosive and ripping, like there is a volcano inside my head that gradually builds up, simmers for a while, and then *bam*. You can't hear anything because the sound is so loud. You can't see anything because the light is so intense. And I'm exploding with it, disintegrating into millions of pieces. Which is fine, because I'd rather be dead than have it keep on going."

At the same clinic there is an old man who suffers from post-herpetic neuralgia. Following an episode of shingles, Mr. H developed recurrent pain down the back of his left leg. *It feels like the leg is on fire*, he tells the doctor. It is so bad that he finds himself instinctively rushing to splash cold water on it.

Knives, hammers, vises, fire. All potential 'weapons used to describe and distinguish pain, which makes it easier for doctors to diagnose and treat their patients. But not everyone is as imaginative as John, Rachel, and Mr. H. And many, especially those who have lived with pain too long, don't even bother trying. They are sick and tired of explaining how they feel to doctors who either don't believe them or never seem to be able to help. For these less forthcoming patients, pain specialists sometimes use the McGill Pain Questionnaire, created in the 1970s by Ronald Melzack and Gil Torgerson. Dissatisfied with primitive pain scales like the mute faces on the

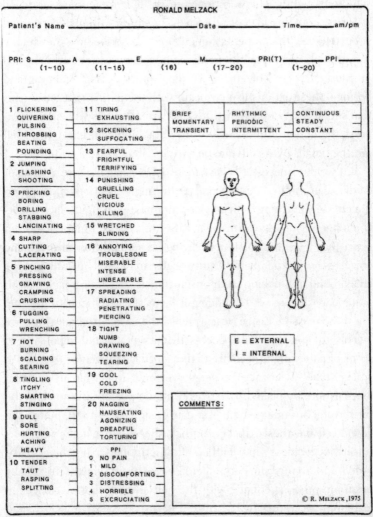

McGILL PAIN QUESTIONNAIRE
RONALD MELZACK

Patient's Name _____ Date _____ Time _____ am/pm

PRI: S _____ A _____ E _____ M _____ PRI(T) _____ PPI _____
    (1–10)   (11–15)   (16)   (17–20)   (1–20)

1 FLICKERING	11 TIRING
QUIVERING	EXHAUSTING
PULSING	12 SICKENING
THROBBING	SUFFOCATING
BEATING	
POUNDING	13 FEARFUL
	FRIGHTFUL
2 JUMPING	TERRIFYING
FLASHING	
SHOOTING	14 PUNISHING
	GRUELLING
3 PRICKING	CRUEL
BORING	VICIOUS
DRILLING	KILLING
STABBING	
LANCINATING	15 WRETCHED
	BLINDING
4 SHARP	
CUTTING	16 ANNOYING
LACERATING	TROUBLESOME
	MISERABLE
5 PINCHING	INTENSE
PRESSING	UNBEARABLE
GNAWING	
CRAMPING	17 SPREADING
CRUSHING	RADIATING
	PENETRATING
6 TUGGING	PIERCING
PULLING	
WRENCHING	18 TIGHT
	NUMB
7 HOT	DRAWING
BURNING	SQUEEZING
SCALDING	TEARING
SEARING	
	19 COOL
8 TINGLING	COLD
ITCHY	FREEZING
SMARTING	
STINGING	20 NAGGING
	NAUSEATING
9 DULL	AGONIZING
SORE	DREADFUL
HURTING	TORTURING
ACHING	
HEAVY	PPI
	0 NO PAIN
10 TENDER	1 MILD
TAUT	2 DISCOMFORTING
RASPING	3 DISTRESSING
SPLITTING	4 HORRIBLE
	5 EXCRUCIATING

BRIEF	RHYTHMIC	CONTINUOUS
MOMENTARY	PERIODIC	STEADY
TRANSIENT	INTERMITTENT	CONSTANT

E = EXTERNAL
I = INTERNAL

COMMENTS:

© R. MELZACK, 1975

"McGill Pain Questionnaire" by Ronald Melzack. *Reprinted with permission from Ronald Melzack.*

chart, the Canadian researchers were convinced that medical care would be greatly improved if patients could only characterize their symptoms better. The questionnaire, in its complete and abridged versions, contains lists of adjectives, organized into categories and subcategories, that patients can choose to describe how they feel.

Although not explicitly mentioned, weapons are clearly implied by most of these adjectives. Burning and shooting, stabbing and boring—these actions usually occur with them: *fires* that burn, *guns* that shoot, *knives* that stab, *drills* that bore. Patients will either compress the action into a single word ("stabbing") or, like John, spell out the details by specifying the weapon, in his case a knife.

But we don't necessarily have to invoke a weapon per se. Angina or cardiac pain is often described as a crushing weight bearing down on the chest by anything from an elephant to a freight train. Rachel talks about her migraines in terms of an active volcano. At times it may even seem that a malevolent human being (as opposed to an inanimate object) is behind our pain, as if the dentist might still be drilling in the area around a throbbing tooth or someone is strangling a patient with pulmonary disease who is finding it increasingly difficult to breathe. For these reasons, Elaine Scarry prefers the more encompassing term "agent" to "weapon" and believes that it's practically impossible to speak of pain without recourse to the "language of agency."

This type of language appears over and over again in personal journals and published narratives of illness. Fanny Burney had the misfortune of undergoing breast cancer surgery in 1810, before the advent of anesthesia. In her journal, she wrote that the pain was "utterly speechless" and "baffled all description." Nonetheless, like Woolf and Styron, she contradicted herself in the next sentence by describing the experience with the help of a weapon no longer in fashion:

So excruciating was the agony . . . when the wound was made and the instrument was withdrawn, the pain seemed undiminished for

the air that suddenly rushed into those delicate parts felt like a
mass of minute but sharp and forked poniards, that were tearing
the edges of the wound.

Toward the end of the same century, Alphonse Daudet was so consumed by the neurological pain of tertiary syphilis—what doctors call
paresthesias and dysesthesias and laypeople call pins and needles—
that he could no longer concentrate on his novels. Like the patients
in Auden's surgical ward, life took place beneath the bandage. Daudet
describes that existence with a series of agency metaphors almost as
exhaustive as the lists found in the McGill Pain Questionnaire:

> Strange aches; great flames of pain furrowing my body, cutting it
> to pieces, lighting it up. . . . Sometimes, on the sole of my foot, an
> incision, a thin one, hair thin. Or a penknife stabbing away beneath
> the big toenail. The torture of the boot! Rats gnawing at the toes
> with very sharp teeth.
>   And amidst all these woes, the sense of a rocket climbing,
> climbing up into your skull, and then exploding there as the climax
> to the show.

More recently another novelist, Reynolds Price, was diagnosed
with cancer of the spinal cord. In his memoir about the experience,
A Whole New Life, Price recalls waking up after the first of many
surgical procedures to remove the recalcitrant tumor:

> The anesthesia wore off enough to let me sense the start of pain
> that would be my constant companion till now. Though it would
> grow and diversify with time, it declared its nature and shape that
> evening. I can still call back that first awareness, the clear sense of
> a white-hot branding iron in the shape of the capital letter "I" held
> against my upper spine from the hairline downward some ten or
> twelve inches and unrelenting.

As the cancer grew and compressed the cord, it left Price in excruciating pain and the branding iron metamorphosed into a living creature:

> *This lethal eel is hid in my spinal cord and will kill me.* From early childhood I'd had a tendency to think in pictures more than words. . . . So once my mind was sober again, I quickly saw the threat as a thing, a visible object; and from the first that object was a dark gray eel embedded live in the midst of my spine.

Even scientists and doctors who are trained to be as direct as possible with language resort to metaphor to convey their pain. Dr. Steven Hsi, a cardiologist who developed a rare and fatal inflammation of his aorta called Takayasu's arteritis, wrote in his memoir, *Closing the Chart*:

> Suddenly, two great claws clamped down on my chest, compressing it with such excruciating pain that I could not breathe.

So despite pain's resistance to language, words often do come, sometimes immediately, in the thick of pain, and sometimes later, after it has passed. And when they come, the words almost exclusively take the form of something or someone acting on our body, forming our core metaphor for the experience.

WEAPONS AND WAR

A more elaborate version of agency occurs in the most common way we speak about illness, what Susan Sontag in *Illness as Metaphor* calls the military metaphor. But instead of the single agent and the more confined confrontations we envision in pain, we often see multiple weapons and battlefronts in illness—in short, a full-scale war, regardless of whether the illness is acute or chronic, life-threatening or less serious. John is fighting appendicitis, Rachel her migraines. An AIDS patient battles the human immunodeficiency virus, another patient the wart virus. In fact, my patient Sandy, who developed rheumatoid arthritis in her teens, often thinks of her entire life in this way. "It's been a constant struggle," she will say, "with some big battles [the joint replacements and lengthy recovery periods] and many smaller ones [getting up in the morning and making breakfast]. The disease is trying to destroy me and I'm doing everything I can just to keep standing. Literally, to keep standing. I realize this sounds like an exaggeration, but the fact is, I'm fighting for my life."

Viewing illness in terms of war is not new. The military metaphor goes at least as far back as the seventeenth century, when John Donne wrote what may be the first pathography. In *Devotions on Emergent Occasions*, Donne speaks of his febrile illness as a heavily armed conflict between rival kingdoms, as war and insurrection. The metaphor became more popular at the end of the nineteenth century, with the advent of germ theory. After scientists such as Koch, Jenner, and Pasteur identified bacteria and viruses as the causes of tuberculosis, cholera, smallpox, and rabies, there was a radical shift in the way people thought about disease. Instead of attributing it to vague internal factors (humors) or even vaguer external ones (miasmas), scientists now had proof that living organisms from the outside world could enter and harm the body. Consequently the vocabulary of illness changed—the professional's as well as the layperson's. Infectious organisms were characterized as foreign or enemy "invaders" that "attacked," "penetrated," and "infiltrated" the body. Illness really *was* a kind of war.

At the same time there were important discoveries in immunology, which meant that the battle would not be lopsided. The body could fight back with white blood cells like the phagocyte, which recognizes the invaders and releases toxins to destroy them. One of the chief goals of medicine became harnessing our own internal forces. We may recall George Bernard Shaw's farcical physician in

The Doctor's Dilemma, who cared less about his tuberculosis patients than about stimulating their immune systems:

> No. I say No. Mr. Dubedat: your moral character is nothing to me. I look at you from a purely scientific view. To me you are simply a field of battle in which an invading army of tubercle bacilli struggle with a force of patriotic phagocytes. Having made a promise to your wife to stimulate those phagocytes, I will stimulate them. And I take no other responsibility.

So illness, which routinely included pain, became conceived of as a war taking place in the body. On one side there were agents and enemies (bacteria and viruses), and on the other defenders (the cells of the immune system). Whichever side proved stronger in a particular case would prevail, resulting in recovery, increased morbidity, or possibly death.

For Susan Sontag, however, the full potential of the military metaphor was not realized until the twentieth century, when it was applied to a particular illness. It was in the language that surrounded cancer that many of its rich nuances would emerge. Cancer cells don't simply multiply, they invade. Then they stealthily track to distant sites in the body, setting up tiny outposts (micrometastases) that cannot be detected. And if they are detected, the cancer cells deviously change uniform (that is, their surface proteins) to evade our immune systems all over again. It is difficult for the body and its defenses to keep up. Most of the time, remission is temporary, as rogue cells inevitably regroup and mount a new offensive. Cancer is a relentless adversary.

Just as descriptions of cancer rely heavily on military terminology, so too do its treatments. In order to bolster the body's immune system, physicians draw from their ever-growing therapeutic arsenals. Chemotherapeutic agents like nitrogen mustard were actually first used as weapons in World War II. In the fight against cancer, however, their purpose is to destroy malignant cells, without, it is hoped, killing the patient's normal cells. Radiation therapy is often discussed in terms of aerial warfare; patients are "bombarded" with toxic rays. And the newest agents in the field continue the trend. The pill Gleevec, a recent breakthrough in the treatment of leukemia, is promoted as a medical "smart bomb" that can obliterate its target with minimal collateral damage.

Inured to the language of their doctors, cancer patients also think and speak militaristically. It would be hard to find a pathography that doesn't envision cancer as a battle or war of sorts. Examples include Joyce Mitchell's *Winning the Chemo Battle* and Cornelius and Kathryn Ryan's *A Private Battle*. Gilda Radner writes in her memoir, *It's Always Something*, that ovarian cancer embroiled her in the battle of her life, "a war against cancer taking place in my own body." In fact, the metaphor has become so pervasive that it has moved beyond the medical setting and become ingrained in the culture at large. Alexander Solzhenitsyn imagines his fictional character in *Cancer Ward* sitting doubled over in bed and sweating with pain, in the midst of a deadly uphill battle:

> The secondaries were tearing his defenses to pieces like tanks, they were hardening his thoracic wall and appearing in the lungs ... The organism was providing no reinforcements, nothing to stop their advance.

And Richard Nixon, a politician, believed that one can only fight like with like and so declared "War on Cancer."

Clearly the military metaphor will remain an enduring part of the vocabulary of illness, in large part because of its resemblance to scientific fact (the biology of infection and malignancy). Yet we must not forget its rhetorical status. Illness is *not* war. Seeing it that way is a metaphor, a fictional *remaking* of illness. As Sontag reminds us, these patently false remakings can have harmful consequences for both individual patients and society as a whole. They contribute to the stigmas associated with disease and can lead us to act against our own interests.

While we should not ignore these consequences, we should emphasize the more benign aspects of the military metaphor. The metaphor provides us with a way to talk and think about events occurring inside the body, events that most of us have limited access to. By linking such events with familiar objects in the external world, as Stephen Dedalus did with the bathroom sink and the roar of the train passing through a tunnel, we can begin to understand and share them with others. Moreover, the particular object chosen in this case, war, is perceived as relevant to the experience of illness not only because of its affinity to scientific fact but also because of its affinity to the language of agency. Cancer patients inevitably feel pain. And in pain they inevitably see weapons that can harm and destroy them—guns and tanks and bombs.

BLURRING THE INSIDE AND THE OUTSIDE

Why always weapons and pain? What makes the connection so automatic? Why is the metaphor so effective? What does it capture about the experience? A logical approach to answering these questions would be to break down the metaphor and consider how well the weapon or agent matches up to the pain.

But there is another way. Before looking at the more complex for clues, we might turn to the more basic—to the very beginnings of language. How is it possible for language to gain a foothold in the realm of private experience in the first place? Conversely, how can something as subjective as pain ever come to be expressed in language, an activity that we engage in with other people and therefore not possibly private? The questions can be posed more ontologically (how does a child learn what pain is?) or more phylogenetically (how might primitive man have learned to communicate pain?). Regardless, we know that in both cases *this does and did indeed happen*—an accomplishment that is truly remarkable. Human beings have managed to create a language that speaks not only about the world outside us, which we share with others (sunsets, birds, flowers), but also about an inside world, which we don't share (love, fear, pain). This language inevitably brings our intimate and solitary selves together into community.

But how?

As Ludwig Wittgenstein explains in his *Philosophical Investigations,* we accomplish this by anchoring language (and meaning, for that matter) in the sharable world, by relying on public or observable criteria. If we want to describe our feeling of love, we do so by speaking through the person or thing we love. And if there is no object, as in the case of pain, then we must invent one, as Stephen Dedalus does. We point outwardly for what we feel inwardly. But before the bathroom sinks and roaring trains and sophisticated weaponry, what might there be to see? What about pain is public and observable?

There are only two possibilities: the *contexts* in which pain occurs and the *behavior* that surrounds it. As we learn early on in life, pain typically follows injury. The sensation occurs when we cut our hand on a sharp object, when we get too close to the fire, when we crash into someone or something. In each case, the environment impinges on the body and causes damage. Second, the sensation typically leads us to behave in certain ways: we scream or cry; we attend to and soothe the injured part of the body; finally, we move away from whatever caused the pain.

Wittgenstein refers to these critical contexts and behaviors surrounding pain as "primitive" and "prelinguistic." Children make the association between how they feel inside and what they see outside *before* or *in the process of* acquiring language, either alone or with the help of a teacher or parent. The only public manifestations of a private experience, these contexts and behaviors form the foundation around which a communal activity such as language arises. A child learns the word "pain" when he learns to connect the sensation with its context (injury) and the resultant behavior (crying, soothing the injured body part, and withdrawing). A child steps onto the fire's ashes, scalds his foot, and cries (and might have watched others do the same). *That's what people call pain*, the child comes to realize. *That's what pain* is.

As time passes, however, and the word becomes a permanent part of the child's vocabulary, it is no longer necessary to emphasize the connection. We don't have to point to an injury to get the message across to another person. Nor do we have to cry or withdraw. Simply saying "I am in pain" implies all that. The contexts and behavior have become internalized. They have shifted to the background, to the unspoken history of language.

Unfortunately, this shifting makes us forget the considerable amount of stage-setting that once took place. To the adult in pain— John in the emergency room, for example, or Rachel J and Mr. H in the pain clinic—the generic word "pain" seems so limited; how much of one's particular experience can it really convey? Very little, we believe. Even when reminded of its history, we are not apt to be satisfied. Fine, we might concede, the contexts and behavior may be important in getting language under way, but they are *not* what pain is. Injury precedes pain and behavior follows pain. But the actual pain, *how it feels*—the blinding light and deafening roar of Rachel's migraine—is left out of the equation. And that's what is most important, that's what we want to communicate to other people.

But is it really left out? Is our shared notion of pain only about contexts and behavior and not about how we feel? No. The felt experience of pain is so intimately bound up with those contexts and behavior that it would be impossible to disentangle them. That is why even in cases when pain doesn't occur in the usual contexts or cause us to behave in the usual ways, *we feel all these things*. Even when there is no visible injury, a broken bone or bloody wound, we feel like there must be some invisible or interior damage. And even when we keep our pain to ourselves, we feel like screaming and withdrawing or running away. All these feelings have been inscribed into our collective notion of pain.

UNRAVELING AGENCY

Still, it remains difficult to believe that so much is compressed into our generic word for pain, which is why we feel the need to decompress it, to spell it out. This is where the agency metaphor comes into play. The agency metaphor brings to the surface what has been stored and lies hidden in the word "pain." It reenacts those prelinguistic settings and behaviors associated with the experience. And the reenactment is organized into a logical sequence, a narrative, with a beginning, middle, and end—a narrative that replaces the blankness and invisibility of pain.

Consider John's abdominal pain. He describes the sudden and sharp sensation as stabbing. It feels as if a knife is penetrating the surface of his belly.

The story would seem to begin with the sharp sensation. But John has learned to process the information by going further back in time, so instead the story begins with an object that *moves toward* him. He imagines a knife, an agent that, like the sharp object, fire, or wall in the prelinguistic contexts of pain, *precedes* the pain.

The story ends with John *moving* in the opposite direction, *away* from the object. He winces and tightens (or pulls back) his belly, a response that corresponds to the prelinguistic behavior that accompanies pain; we scream and withdraw from the sharp object, fire, or wall *after* we feel the pain because it has hurt us and we don't want the hurt to continue.

Finally, John connects the beginning and ending of the story by inferring a middle—namely, injury to the body—that provides a causal explanation for the sensation. An agent moves toward us, makes damaging contact with the body (injury), and causes us pain, so we move away from it.

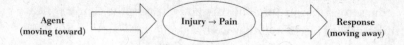

Agent (moving toward) → Injury → Pain → Response (moving away)

Unraveling the language of agency, we find that the metaphor brings together the many different layers that make up this complex experience. Psychologists and philosophers have always found it difficult to categorize pain: Is it a sensation or perception? A form of behavior? An emotional or cognitive state? The truth is that pain is all of these. Clearly it involves having a sensation. But that sensation cannot be separated from our responses to the sensation: behavioral responses (withdrawing), emotional responses (crying), and cognitive ones (inferring a cause). Everything happens, or at least seems to happen, simultaneously.

Most important, the metaphor captures how pain feels, its phenomenology. It captures what Elaine Scarry calls the defining quality of the experience, its aversiveness (derived from the Latin *avertere*, "to turn away from"). While other sensations can be viewed positively, neutrally, or negatively, pain is

a pure physical experience of negation, an immediate sensory rendering of "against," of something being against one, and of something one must be against. Even though it occurs within oneself, it is at once identified as "not oneself," "not me," as something so alien that it must right now be gotten rid of.

This aversiveness originates directly from the prelinguistic contexts and behavior surrounding pain and is vividly dramatized in the metaphor of agency, in its dual and opposing movements.

On the one hand, pain's aversiveness is the feeling of "something being against one." We feel as if there must be an agent moving against (and threatening) the body: Burney's poniards, Daudet's penknife, Price's eel, John's knife, Rachel's volcano, Mr. H's fire. Or, more elaborately (in the military version), an enemy or alien force marches against and attacks the body's interior, like the advance of the secondaries in Solzenhitsyn's novel, tearing the cancer patient's defenses to pieces as if they were tanks.

At the same time, pain's aversiveness is the feeling "of something one must be against." We desperately want to move away from the agent moving toward us. Whether or not we actually move—John, for example, moves only the muscles of his belly (guarding it against another attack of pain)—we feel like doing so. Or perhaps more accurately, we feel like running away—Rachel wants to be so far from the blinding lights and deafening roar of her migraines that at times she'd like to disappear or die. If we can't run from an interior threat like cancer, then perhaps we can jettison the alien invader, getting rid of it by whatever means possible.

Finally, we feel the need to connect these opposing movements. It is impossible to have pain—an experience that threatens to obliterate us and everything else in the world—without wanting an explanation. *Why is this happening to me?* ask John and Rachel. *What is causing it?* The agency metaphor provides an answer: the knife or volcanic explosion that moves against them, that will ultimately strike their bodies and produce pain, and that they should run away from. In pain, we feel that something is against us and that we must be against *because* that something is hurting us—hurting us in both senses we ascribe to the word, causing injury *and* pain.

By returning to the origins of language, on the one hand, and then dissecting a more complex form of language (the agency metaphor), on the other, we have inched closer to the phenomenology of pain, what it actually feels like. Remarkably, we find that our feelings are not as personal and private as we may have thought, that they can be represented in language. All this is possible because our feelings, just like our word "pain," arise from and remain connected to certain public and observable phenomena. Pain is the feeling that we want to scream (even if we don't), the feeling that we want to run away (even if we don't), the feeling that there is something against us that we should run from (even if there is not), and the feeling that all this is happening because something is damaging our bodies (even if there is no damage).

INJURY AND PAIN

We saw that injury plays an important role in how pain language gets started. We also saw that injury is an important component of the phenomenology of pain. So it shouldn't be surprising that injury appears in the most common way we talk about pain, the language of agency. Yet that appearance is far less prominent than the objects we envision moving toward us and our desire to move away from them. While we always see weapons in pain, we don't always see injuries. They typically lie beneath the surface.

Nonetheless, injury is the linchpin of agency. It binds the narrative together. We feel pain because we assume there has been damage to our body and want to avoid further damage (and further pain). Pain, in fact, has become practically synonymous with injury:

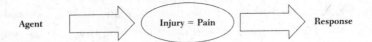

That is why, of all possible agents, we gravitate toward the weapon. The weapon is effective at representing pain because its sole function is to injure; it too is synonymous with injury. For this same reason, the military metaphor is effective at representing cancer. As much as politicians might claim otherwise, the purpose of war is to injure and kill as many people as possible—hence the use of guns, bombs, and missiles. The only difference in cancer is that the battlefield, with all its carnage and pain, is situated within a single human body.

But while injury is necessary to metaphors and narratives of pain, *it is not necessary to actual pain*. The complexity of pain, discussed earlier in terms of its sensational, emotional, and cognitive dimensions, also extends to the biological. Although we used to think of pain as a warning bell that tells the brain when the body has been injured (once again Descartes is held to blame), we now know that this is not true. The perception of pain—perception implying that pain is not passively experienced but must be actively processed by the brain—is influenced by a variety of factors, including genetics, neuroanatomy, emotions, and expectations. That is why different people don't experience the same pain (quantitatively or qualitatively) when they get stuck with a needle; why people of different cultures don't experience pain equivalently; why some people experience no pain despite very serious damage to the body and others experience excruciating pain with no damage; why people born with certain genetic defects or who have specific injuries to the brain can have completely abnormal responses to injury; and why it can be difficult to distinguish between physical and mental pain. The bottom line is that pain doesn't follow injury in a strict one-to-one correspondence; they are *not* synonymous and are on occasion completely detachable.

Injury ≠ Pain

The same, however, cannot be said for the way we think and talk of pain. As we just saw, only by connecting pain with injury is it possible for language to gain a foothold in the realm of private experience. Initially we point to occasions when pain follows a visible injury. The connection is reinforced over time, so that even in instances where there is no visible injury, we assume there must be some internal, invisible injury. Inevitably pain and injury become inseparable in our minds; we cannot think of pain without thinking of injury or without thinking of agents and weapons and war, all of which cause injury.

Injury, then, is as much a *metaphor* of pain as it is an actual biological fact about pain. Even physicians, who have traditionally been most committed to the biomedical account of pain equating the two, are beginning to recognize the metaphorical status of injury. In 1979 a committee formed by the International Association for the Study of Pain agreed on the following definition:

Pain is the unpleasant sensory and emotional experience *associated with actual or potential tissue damage, or described in terms of such damage.* (my italics)

Only by acknowledging this point can we begin to validate the pain of patients with chronic pain syndromes such as fibromyalgia (where there may be no injury) and those who suffer psychologically, like Joan Didion (in grief) and William Styron (in depression). Regardless of the presence of actual tissue damage, we intimate such damage and describe pain *in terms of* such damage. For example, the psychiatrist and patient Kay Redfield Jamison speaks in her memoir, *An Unquiet Mind*, of the "terrible wounds" exacted by her manic-depressive episodes, which often took months to heal. And Toni Morrison places a horrific wound on the back of Sethe in her novel *Beloved*. The dense thicket of scar tissue in the form of a chokecherry tree is a visible and permanent record of the pain— both physical and emotional—that Sethe suffered as a slave. We can't help but shudder and put our hands over our mouth when we read about the wound, just as Sethe's mother-in-law, Baby Suggs, does when she sees it for the first time. Morrison's image makes it possible to convey, even if incompletely, Sethe's pain, which, in the author's words—and in the experience of many sufferers—is "unspeakable."

7

Literary Agency

> The pain was excruciating and violent. . . . It came
> in long ocean rollers. He couldn't get on the other
> side of it.
>
> —ANNIE PROULX, "The Mud Below"

The agency metaphor is an exceptionally good metaphor. It brings to the surface what has been internalized in our generic word for pain. But there is a danger in relying exclusively on a single metaphor. When used over and over again, the language of agency loses its suggestiveness and powers of illumination. Too often we say a pain is stabbing; we no longer see the knife that the metaphor should evoke. We begin to feel that it doesn't convey much more about the experience than the word "pain."

Therefore we must find ways to revive our older metaphors and continually create new ones. Our best chance at finding such novel approaches would be to change venues—to move from the emergency room to the literary world, from John's stabbing pains to the festering wound on Sethe's back in *Beloved* and the ocean rollers that come at Annie Proulx's character and can't be avoided—for revival and novelty are in a sense what literature, and indeed art in general, is all about: they work to make us see and think about things we ordinarily fail to see, thereby offering us a view of reality that can often be more "real" and revealing than reality itself. Literature accomplishes this primarily through the manipulation of space and time. In the real world, especially the world of the hospital, everything happens so quickly that we barely have time to register all the details, let alone arrange them in meaningful patterns. The literary world pauses events, enabling us to see things we might otherwise have missed and to distill the essence of an experience. The prime function of art, writes the philosopher Susanne Langer, "is to make the felt tensions of life, from the diffused somatic tonus of vital sense to the highest intensities of mental and emotional experience, stand still to be looked at." Through the arresting mechanism of artifice, literature can shed light on the experience of pain as well as on the language we use to communicate pain. Writers are drawn to the agency metaphor just like the rest of us, yet they are generally intolerant of cliché and dead metaphor. They will work to elaborate and stretch the metaphor in ways that may enhance our understanding of pain's aversiveness and perhaps even point out features we hadn't previously recognized.

The literary works we will examine are mainly short stories written by nineteenth- and twentieth-century writers, including Leo Tolstoy, Guy de Maupassant, Stephen Crane, and Jack London. They are all overtly about pain, which, according to Virginia Woolf, makes them relatively unique in literature. Additionally, the pain depicted in the stories is caused by extreme weather conditions (in particular the cold) rather than by common diseases that are already saturated with metaphor, such as cancer and AIDS. This offers us an opportunity to watch how a seemingly neutral entity is transformed into a destructive agent. Finally, these stories are exceptional recreations of the felt experience of suffering in general, of the epoché that pain brings about. Whether in the desolate wilderness of the Yukon or Caucasus or alone amid the endless expanse of the Atlantic Ocean, the protagonists find themselves isolated from civilization—a literal rendering of Auden's surgical patients, who only seem to be as "remote as plants."

Yet while they emphasize the solitary dimension of pain, the stories also emphasize its communal aspect, because the protagonist (or the author on his or her behalf) is *responding* to the crisis. More accurately, the stories reflect the dialectic present in the crisis of pain, a dialectic that ranges from the solitary, personal, and private nature of the experience to the communal, social, and public meanings we ascribe to it. It is precisely because these texts are situated at the boundary between these two poles, waiting for the moment when words emerge from the silence, that we as readers cannot help but feel present at a birthing point of language.

PAIN AS THREAT

Jack London holds a special place in literature. Unlike many writers, he not only imagined what he wrote about but actually lived it. Most of his stories and novels take place in the frigid, inhospitable Yukon Territory of northwestern Canada. There London and the characters in his stories braved the elements in their quest for glory and gold. Many of these adventures resulted in a great deal of pain—London, we know, suffered from scurvy, alcoholism, liver and kidney disease, and depression—which the writer became adept at conveying.

Mason, from the short story "The White Silence," is one of these adventurers. He is in the midst of long trek through the Northlands with his wife and a companion. They have another two hundred miles to go. The temperature is sixty-five degrees below zero, their food is running out, and the sled dogs are tiring. It is at this point that Mason stops to tie his shoes. The timing couldn't be worse, for Mason is standing beneath a giant pine tree, weighed down by old age and snow. The accident is sudden and swift. The tree gives way and crushes him.

Mason doesn't die instantly. He languishes for days in what must be excruciating pain. Yet we hear nothing of his pain, because Mason is so mangled that he can hardly speak, except for "an occasional moan." And even if he were able to speak, chances are that he wouldn't. What could he say that would make sense of what just happened, that might convey how he feels? Nothing, we are led to believe by the narrator, who tells us of the stoic ways of the people raised in this region, taught from early on the "futility of words."

Mason is our prototypical sufferer. He is like the man in the Munch painting, alone and unable to vocalize except for inarticulate moans; his pain is incommunicable. Remarkably, London's story of Mason radically changes this. While one set of observers, Mason's wife and companion, is walled off from the sufferer, another set of observers is not. We, as readers of the story, feel as if we understand, albeit incompletely, what Mason is experiencing, for while Mason remains silent, the narrator speaks on his behalf.

From the outset, the narrator prepares us for the pain to come by identifying an agent prior to the accident. There is a part of nature, he says, that has separated itself from the rest and can no longer be thought of as a backdrop against which the travelers journey. It has come to possess the capacity to harm living things—the trees, the sled dogs, even human beings. The narrator gives this part of nature a name. He calls it the White Silence:

> Nature has many tricks wherewith she convinces man of his finity—the ceaseless flow of the tides, the fury of the storm, the shock of the earthquake, the long roll of heaven's artillery—but the most tremendous, the most stupefying of all, is the passive phase of the White Silence. All movement ceases, the sky clears, the heavens are as brass; the slightest whisper seems sacrilege, and man becomes timid, affrighted at the sound of his own voice. Sole speck of life journeying across the ghostly wastes of a dead world, he trembles at his audacity, realizes that his is a maggot's life, nothing more.

When tragedy finally strikes, it doesn't seem to matter that "little is said." The reader already has a sense of the tremendous hostile force that has crushed Mason. We see (and almost hear) the White

Silence, the agent that will stand in for the subsequent pain and objectify Mason's feelings—that there is a something against him and that there is a something which he must be against. In this way, London communicates what his character cannot.

London's portrayal of the Silence as an agent also enhances our understanding of the experience. The metaphor responds to the "Why?" of pain. Though not the direct cause (it is responsible through its effect on the aging tree), the White Silence is identified as possessing *the capacity to cause pain and damage*; it is identified as a threat. Unfortunately, Mason doesn't benefit from the knowledge. It's the narrator who understands, not him, with only the reader standing to benefit. We would surely be more mindful of the deadly traps that the Silence has set for us. We sense, however, that London too wishes for a different, more sympathetic ending to his story. If only Mason were able to see what the narrator sees, then perhaps he would not have stopped where he did.

Part of Mason's problem, like that of many of London's characters who suffer in the Yukon, is a lack of imagination. The warning signs are right in front of him; he just doesn't heed them. The other problem is the subtlety of the particular agent. Because of its silence and passivity, the White Silence remains vague and abstract. In order for us to recognize its threat more clearly, the agent must become animated; it must literally be able to *move* against its victim. This is the case with the cold air in Tolstoy's story "Lost on the Steppe," which "forces its way through the opening" of a character's coat sleeves. Finding himself lost in a snowstorm, Tolstoy's traveler feels progressively colder. He is also consumed by anxiety as he recalls the story of a group of men who recently froze to death. To objectify these feelings, he transforms the cold into an agent that moves against his body: "My nose and cheeks felt as if they were freezing, more frequently the draught of cold air insinuated itself under my shuba."

Guy de Maupassant uses this kind of imagery in "The First Snowfall." Like Tolstoy's man (and unlike Mason), the female protagonist of his story is sensitive to the threat posed by the environment. She has lived most her life in southern France and now, because of an arranged marriage, suddenly finds herself in the colder, more inhospitable wintry landscape of Normandy. The woman feels the cold in "the marrow of her bones" and believes that prolonged exposure will cause great harm. But when she tells her husband, he ignores her. One is reminded of Scarry's insight that while being in pain can be equated with certainty, observing someone in pain can be equated with skepticism. To say "I am cold and it hurts" may not be enough. The woman must find a more effective way to express her pain.

She does so by objectifying the cold as an enemy that moves against her body, hovering over the skin and threatening entry:

> Sharper, more penetrating still than the year before, the cold made her suffer, continually . . . icy puffs seemed to slip down her back and to penetrate between the flesh and her underclothing. And she shook from head to foot. Innumerable currents of air appeared to have taken up their abode in the apartment, living, crafty currents of air as cruel as enemies. She encountered them every moment, they were incessantly buffeting, sometimes on the face, sometimes on the neck, with their treacherous, frozen breath.

By imagining the cold air as a living entity—an agent that is "incessantly buffeting" her—the woman converts her inner sensation of being cold and her fears about prolonged exposure into an external picture (in words). The metaphor enables the woman to convey her feelings to others; the reader can almost see the cold and empathizes with her. It also helps her to clarify those feelings. She now has a better sense of what she's up against and responds accordingly. Like Tolstoy's freezing man, who "bundles up tightly" to stave off the insinuating cold air, Maupassant's woman repeatedly asks her husband for a furnace. But the husband doesn't see the hostile trajectory of the cold air and denies her requests. It is only when the danger is recognized that one can begin to protect oneself and others.

These literary examples underscore a critical element in the felt experience of pain that has been alluded to but not yet clearly defined. In "The White Silence," the narrator describes the environment as an agent so that the reader can anticipate a painful event. Similarly, Tolstoy's man and Maupassant's woman picture the cold as threatening them. The focus is on the agent's potential to cause pain rather than actual pain; at the level of narrative, this is called foreshadowing. Like the gun or other weapon prominently displayed early on in a Hollywood thriller, foreshadowing provides dramatic suspense and tension. But that same kind of suspense and tension is occurring in another narrative, one that unfolds not on the pages of a story or in the consciousness of the reader but in the very interior of the person who suffers, in the felt experience of pain itself. Pain registers a lot like foreshadowing. It is as much an immediate, present-tense phenomenon as it is the anticipation, anxiety, and uncertainty of what the future holds; it involves the having of pain as much as it does the threat of having pain or the threat of experiencing more pain or more severe pain.

The fact that pain includes an element of threat should be self-evident. After all, from a biological or evolutionary standpoint, this is one of its primary functions. Pain is a warning signal that the body is in danger and that demands an appropriate response. It tells us to withdraw our hand from the flame, to take cover from the cold, to rest the leg when a bone has been broken. In instances when the signal is missing, the consequences are often catastrophic. Children who are born without the ability to feel pain and adults with acquired abnormalities that can occur in diabetes and leprosy have significantly shortened life spans. Because they can't feel pain, they don't recognize threats in the environment, which lead to repeated injury, infection, and ultimately premature death.

Yet despite the obvious, we find it difficult to think of pain in both actual and potential terms (just as we find it difficult to think of the

mind and body in the same breath). Pain, we feel, is the body reporting an injury. The anticipation or threat of injury, though, registers
only in the mind and must be classified with other psychological
experiences, like anxiety and depression. Maupassant's woman suffers pain from the cold *and* from anguish about the future. Shouldn't
they be treated as two distinct experiences?

We have seen that this distinction makes no sense. Researchers
have clearly demonstrated that pain routinely extends beyond the
strictly physical, as it does in chronic pain syndromes like lower
back pain and fibromyalgia, where no organic damage is detected.
Over a century ago Freud pointed out the intense pain often present in conditions such as grief and depression. Back in the pain
clinic, Rachel J tells her doctor that the aura preceding her
migraines (a series of visual sensations that by themselves aren't
painful) is almost as painful as the actual migraines; the anticipation of what will come is so unbearable that she prays for the headache to start. In a similar vein, Lucy Grealy writes in her cancer
memoir, *Autobiography of a Face*, that the pain of being deformed
and ugly was far greater (and more threatening) than any pain she
experienced from surgery or chemotherapy.

The common denominator in all of these instances is not tissue
damage but a shared underlying structure. Pain, as we defined it, is
an all-consuming interior experience that *threatens to destroy everything except itself*—language, other people, the world, and ultimately
the self. This shared structure of an overwhelming threat gives rise
to shared representations. In the thick of his depression, Styron uses
the agency metaphor just as Daudet and Fanny Burney do; he felt,
he writes, as if he were being "suffocated" and "drowned," as if there
were a "howling tempest" battering his brain. Similarly the Mexican
painter Frida Kahlo paints the emotional pain arising from her infer-
tility and her marital problems in the same way she depicts the neurological pain from her damaged spinal cord; the former quite
literally pierces her heart.

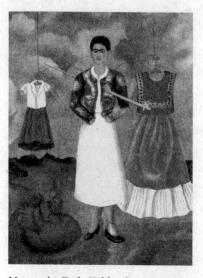

Memory by Frida Kahlo. © 2009 *Banco
de Mexico Diego Rivera Frida Kahlo*
Museums Trust, Mexico, D.F. / Artists
Rights Society (ARS).

A pioneer in the medical humanities, Dr. Eric Cassell is sensitive
to the continuity between physical and mental pain. He believes
such sensitivity has eluded contemporary medicine, causing it consistently to fall short in caring for patients. Pain isn't just confined to
the present or to the body but extends through time and over the
person as a whole. Occurring when "an impending destruction of
the person is perceived, it continues until the threat of disintegra-
tion has passed or until the integrity of the person has been restored."
While Cassell calls this extension of pain "suffering," I would argue
that we don't need another category to account for it. "Pain" can and
should incorporate these extra elements.

Earlier we emphasized the "corporal engulfment" (Scarry) that
one experiences in pain—that in pain there's nothing but *the body in
pain*. But what should become clear, especially in light of Cassell's

comments and our examples of literary agency, is that the fracturing of the body's integrity in pain has its counterpart in the fracturing of the self; as the intactness of the body dissolves, so too does the intactness of the person as a whole. We might say, then, that the epoché of pain involves not only a bracketing of the world (putting it out of play, in Merleau-Ponty's words), but a bracketing of the person. Pain literally says—screams in fact, as it does to Tolstoy's character in "Lost on the Steppe," freezing in the Caucasus and thinking about his fellow travelers who recently froze to death—*SOS . . . Fear for your life . . . You, body and soul, are in danger of being obliterated*. It screamed this to William Styron, who when suffocating in the grip of depression recalled Camus's suicide, and to Joan Didion, who was unable to think rationally after her husband died. A large part of pain's painfulness, as Cassell astutely observes, is the uncertainty of the future, the real possibility of extinction—as in the waiting of Denise Levertov's poem "Divorcing":

> We were Siamese twins.
> Our blood's not sure if it can circulate,
> Now that we are cut apart.
> Something in each of us is waiting
> To see if we can survive severed.

By now it should be clear that foreshadowing an agent (describing it before pain occurs) isn't merely a narrative device. It also captures an essential aspect of pain: the feeling of impending destruction—of John's knife, say, moving toward him and threatening his life. And this feeling can literally be spoken of as a warning signal, one that has its parallel in the biological function of pain, because pain is indeed a signal that alerts us to imminent danger and urges us to avoid that danger at all costs.

We will call this the signaling aspect of the agency metaphor. When seen as moving against the body, the cold portrayed as an agent objectifies the perception of a threat, and in doing so *commu-*

nicates that perception to the sufferer (the characters in the story) as well as to an outside observer (the reader of the story). We might imagine ways to enhance this signal, to articulate it more clearly and thereby ensure that the message is understood. This is precisely what a clever writer like Tolstoy does when he makes the environment convey its threat not just tacitly (by moving against his character) but also quite literally (by acquiring a voice). Lost, freezing, isolated, Tolstoy's man hears the wind first "whistle" and then "wail." As the storm worsens, the wind speaks in more ominous tones: it begins to "howl." In this way the agent *announces* its destructive potential and the man, recognizing the threat, has a chance to protect himself.

We begin to detect a progression in the language of agency. The more elaborate the metaphor, the better it is at communicating pain. London's unfortunate character is oblivious to the threat hovering over him (which the author clearly conveys to his readers) because the Silence moves against Mason more figuratively than literally. By contrast, Maupassant's woman identifies the cruel currents of air moving toward her; she realizes that she must act to avoid further harm (by getting a furnace) but is prevented by her husband. Finally, in Tolstoy's story, the cold communicates on its own—it acquires a voice and speaks to the man.

What is fascinating about this final conceit is that the agent's acquisition of speech comes just as the sufferers lose their own ability to speak. Earlier we suggested that our stories of extremity can be taken as metaphors of the crisis of pain enacted every day in hospital wards across the country. London's and Tolstoy's characters find themselves at the outermost fringes of civilization. Because language provides a means of self-extension—a means of moving beyond the self and toward others—it offers a way out of the crisis. But pain, in its adamant resistance to language, appears to obstruct this escape route when it is most desperately needed. Worse, as Elaine Scarry observes, pain actively destroys language, "bringing about a reversion to a state anterior to language, to the sound and cries a human makes before language is learned." That is why Munch's depiction of the scream that goes unheard is such a powerful representation of the experience.

If these stories can be viewed as metaphors of what pain accomplishes, the agents within them can be viewed as metaphors of how it does so. The agents become instruments of pain, acting out its invisible machinations. Like pain, Tolstoy's wind diligently works to destroy language. We are told that it "tears" the voice from the narrator's mouth as he tries to speak—the narrator, who, we mustn't forget, is called upon to convey his experience to us readers—and "carries it in a twinkling far from him." Later on, as the situation becomes more dire, the narrator announces that "we have no voices left." Besides speech, the agent takes away other routes of escaping the "ferocious inwardness" of pain. Tolstoy's wind is said "to cut" his character's eyes, blinding him to the outside world. This shattering of language and perception underscores the all-consuming nature of pain, its threat to destroy *everything* except itself.

The acquisition of speech by the agent, however, serves to redress the extreme insularity of pain. Whether formulated by a person in pain or by a beneficent author on his behalf—or even perhaps by the body itself, when it speaks to Rachel (and other migraine and epilepsy patients) in the language of the aura—the objectification of pain via agency is truly expressive, addressing the most urgent concerns of the sufferer. Because a character has difficulty speaking or perceiving the threat posed by the environment, the agent is made to announce its own presence; the voice lost by the sufferer is gained by the agent. And inasmuch as this act of worldmaking is a response to crisis, it is inherently pragmatic. A sign is effective only if it can *signify*. That Tolstoy's man and Maupassant's woman respond appropriately, and that a reader of these stories senses the urgency of their situations, testify to the effectiveness, or *significance*, of the agency metaphor.

The waves that threaten the survivors of a shipwreck in Stephen Crane's famous short story "The Open Boat" may be even more articulate than Tolstoy's wind. For the four men in the battered dinghy, floating in the middle of a raging ocean, the world about them continues to dwindle until there is practically nothing except the waves:

> None of them knew the color of the sky. Their eyes glanced level
> and were fastened on the waves that swept toward them.

Because the waves possess the potential to harm, they are represented as agents. Like Maupassant's icy whiffs, Crane's waves move against the men ("the tall black waves swept forward") and do so constantly (they "continued their impetuous swooping at the dinghy"). Additionally, since the men can't see very much and since speech becomes too precarious—even the subtle movements of their facial muscles can tip the fragile dinghy—they must be made to see and hear the threat of the waves. Crane helps them by giving the agent a voice that serves both to announce and to substantiate its threat:

> There was a preparatory and long growl in [the waves'] speech . . .
> the tall black waves swept in a most sinister silence, save for an
> occasional subdued growl of a crest.

Before there is any actual contact between ocean and man, Crane conveys to his reader the potential for such contact (and the anguish accompanying it) that his characters feel at every moment.

The story is exceptionally illustrative because it calls attention to its fictional status. Framed as being written long after the event by one of the survivors (the title's subscript is "A Tale Intended to be after the Fact"), it attempts to convey how the men felt *at the time of crisis*. Naturally the narrator turns to the agency metaphor. But there are two instances when the narrator, safe and secure in his writing study, interrupts his story. In both instances he abruptly changes perspective, removing himself from the confines of the dinghy and trying to imagine the scene from his present vantage point—a perspective that enables him to see not only the waves but the entire panorama:

Viewed from a balcony, the whole thing would doubtlessly have been weirdly picturesque.

It was probably splendid. It was probably glorious, this play of the free sea, wild with lights of emerald and white and amber.

As an observer of pain, separated by time and space, the survivor begins to see the ocean more dispassionately, devoid of the potential for harm; indeed, he says, it must have been a glorious spectacle to behold.

Not so when he was in the boat. Then there was nothing to behold—nothing but the waves (and the pain; they are interchangeable) that growl ferociously at the men and threaten to destroy them.

PAIN AS FORCE

When used primarily to represent a threat, the signaling capacity of the agent (moving against the sufferer) is emphasized. This is most effectively done when the agent is pictured as hovering over the body and threatening entry (in the case of Maupassant's woman and Tolstoy's man) and when it announces its hostility (to Crane's survivors).

But when the focus shifts from the threat of pain to actual pain, from what might happen to what is happening, the metaphor must also shift. When the agent signals pain, it moves *toward* the body. When the agent inflicts pain, it must move *into* the body. The resulting collision will be meaningful, in the sense that it is perceived as the cause of pain, only if the agent possesses a substantial force.

We can think of force in abstract terms, as we do in physics, where force is equivalent to an object of a certain mass moving at a constant rate of velocity. But for contemporary thinkers like Mark Johnson, who believe that consciousness is embodied (that we think with and through our bodies), we learn about force in everyday experiences—when we compete on the football field or try to make headway in a storm. Eventually we recognize a pattern or underlying structure in these experiences. In what Johnson calls an imaginative schema, a force might involve a moving object (a running back with the ball) that encounters a second object (a tackling linebacker); there is a collision; and the degree of impact, or force, depends on the size of the running back and how fast he is moving.

The key element in both versions is the physical dimension of the moving object, its bodily aspect (Johnson) or its mass (physics). And this physicality is central not only to how we think about force but also to how we talk about force. In *The Body in the Mind*, Johnson cites an old newspaper report on the British invasion of the Falklands to make his point:

> The Argentine air force launched a *massive* attack on the British fleet. One frigate was *heavily* damaged, but only *light* casualties were suffered by British sailors. The Argentines paid a *heavy* toll in downed aircraft.

In a quick reading of the passage, the italicized adjectives and adverb might appear as ordinary (i.e., literal) descriptors used to indicate extent or quantity; "massive" and "heavy" indicate a large quantity, "light" a small one. But with some reflection, we notice that they are also metaphors that point to the physical properties of terms like "casualty," "toll," and "damage"—properties that, while important to their meanings, we may not be conscious of. The casualties are light not only because there aren't many dead soldiers but also because the small *body* count doesn't weigh that much.

Good journalists are aware of these subtleties, of what makes communication most effective. If the writer of the war report wants his readers to appreciate the force of the Argentine attack, he will instinctively refer to its physical dimension—it was a *massive* attack that *heavily* damaged the frigate. Without the attention to weight, the attack couldn't possibly have such dire consequences; it becomes less plausible and easier to dismiss. Similarly, a writer using the agency metaphor to represent a painful collision between the environment and his character will emphasize the agent's force; the agent that is moving against the human body (velocity) has to have sufficient bulk (mass) in order for the ensuing pain to be taken seriously; colliding with a Mack truck will surely produce more pain than colliding with a stuffed animal.

Language too, as Scarry observes, can possess force—not merely what the words stand for but the words in themselves. If it has the power to act on and alter the material world—and surely we hope it does—then language must be able to signify forcefully. It too must be capable of "registering in its own contours the contours and weight of the material world."

Thomas Hardy understands the importance of making language substantial when faced with the task of representing the wind, which has no visible material presence, as a destructive agent in *The Woodlanders*. In the novel, Hardy's heroine, Grace, marries the town doctor instead of Giles, the simple woodsman she is in love with. But when she discovers that her husband has been unfaithful, she runs off to Giles's hut in the woods to be with him. The weather is stormy and worsening by the minute. While Grace is safe in the hut, Giles is nowhere to be found. Setting the scene for what will follow (foreshadowing), Hardy paints the wind as an agent:

> The wind grew more violent, and as the storm went on it was difficult to believe that no opaque body, but only an invisible colourless thing, was trampling and climbing over the roof, making branches creak, springing out of the trees upon the chimney, popping its head into the flue, and shrieking and blaspheming at every corner of the walls. As in the grisly story, the assailant was a spectre which could be felt but not seen.

The wind pushes the *hut*, it bends and displaces *trees*, objects that have a substantial material presence. But how can the wind, the invisible wind, exert such force? Only if, despite all appearances to the contrary, as Hardy tells us, it too has a substantial presence, a presence that *makes itself felt* through its effect on the hut and trees. But the wind can also harm the living. As it happens, Giles lies just a few yards away from the hut, exposed and vulnerable. He has been sick, and the storm is now literally killing him. Although Grace is unaware of Giles's proximity and condition—she wonders whether the sound she hears in the distance is someone's cough or the howl of the wind—Hardy and his readers are acutely aware, and for this reason the wind must be seen as an agent, one that can destroy both things and people:

> Sometimes a bough from an adjoining tree was swayed so low as to smite the roof in the manner of a gigantic hand smiting the mouth of an adversary, to be followed by a trickle of rain, as blood from the wound. To all this weather Giles must be more or less exposed; how much she [Grace] did not know.

While Hardy calls attention to the difficulty of representing an agent that can injure the human body but cannot be seen, London devises a strategy that overcomes this difficulty in his story "The Heathen." In order to convey the pain that his character experiences in the face of a gale-force wind, London enhances the wind's physical presence. On a journey to the South Pacific, the sailors on the *Petite Jeanne* find themselves in the middle of a powerful hurricane. The wind that previously assisted them by pushing against the sails of their ship now begins to push and drive against their bodies, and does so with a force that is impossible to describe:

> No; it is beyond me. Language may be adequate to express the ordinary conditions of life, but it cannot possibly express any of the conditions of so enormous a blast of wind. It would have been better had I stuck to my original intention of not attempting a description.

The inability to articulate the force of the wind recalls the familiar response of the patient (*You can't imagine how I feel*) and Woolf's comment that the language quickly runs dry in pain. It is not merely the nature of the wind that creates these semantic difficulties. What is difficult to convey is how much the wind hurts and what that hurt feels like. London responds by magnifying the material nature of the wind:

> One could not face the wind and live. It was a monstrous thing, and the most monstrous thing about it was that it increased and continued to increase.
>
> Imagine countless millions and billions of tons of sand. Imagine this sand tearing along at ninety, a hundred, a hundred and twenty, or any other number of miles per hour. Imagine, further, this sand to be invisible, impalpable, yet to retain all the weight and density of sand. Do all this, and you may get a vague inkling of what the wind was like.
>
> Perhaps sand is not the right comparison. Consider it mud, invisible, impalpable, but heavy as mud . . .

Previously the force of the wind on the sails of the boat was more helpful than harmful and didn't cause the sailors much thought. But when it begins to inflict pain, the wind cannot be ignored; it must be seen as an agent that exerts tremendous force. Initially this transformation is problematic because an invisible, impalpable entity like the wind doesn't appear substantial enough—that is, both massive and believable enough—to wreak such damage. London resolves the problem by making the wind visible and palpable, picturing it as made up of millions of particles, each particle bearing the density of sand and then mud.

London's description with its attention to weight recalls the language of cardiac patients in the emergency room. Here too there is nothing to see; the pain of angina is caused by compromised blood flow to the heart. So patients instinctively invoke an agent: *There is an object pressing down on my chest*, they will say; *that object is heavy;*

a big, heavy box; no, bigger, a car perhaps; better yet, a truck or a freight train. Only by imagining this series of ever-enlarging objects can patients begin to convey and legitimize their pain, both to themselves and to their doctors, who also can't see it.

A hurricane is at the center of another short story by London, "The House of Mapui." This time it sets down on a small island, practically obliterating everything and every person residing there. One inhabitant, as he struggles against the surging winds and witnesses the devastation around him, tries to make sense of what is happening. *How could mere air or water cause so much pain?* he asks himself. Only if it were much more massive than it appears, so massive and dense that you could grasp it as if it were a cliff or a wall:

> The wind was no longer air in motion. He had a feeling that he could reach into it and tear it out in chunks as one might do with the meat in the carcass of a steer; that he could seize hold of the wind and hang on to it as a man might hang on to the face of a cliff.

The water too—it must also be a wall, a "wall without end":

> A frightful wall of water caught [the Mormon church], tilted it, and flung it against half a dozen cocoanut trees. The bunches of human fruit fell like ripe cocoanuts. The subsiding wave showed them on the ground, some lying motionless, others squirming and writhing. They reminded him of ants.

At the same time, the man diminishes the material presence of his fellow sufferers, envisioning them as fruit and ants—a strategy that captures yet another element of the experience of pain. While pain is always enlarging, the sufferer is always shrinking (being consumed). *That freight train bearing down on my increasingly vulnerable chest will surely crush me,* believes the cardiac patient. *Mount Etna erupting in my fragile head will obliterate me in no time,* believes Rachel. *I am no match for the monstrous storms of depression,* believes

Styron, *not in my weakened state*. Pain, the longer it goes on, reduces, consumes, and threatens to erase.

We experience different kinds of contact with other types of pain that can also be represented by the agency metaphor. In addition to contact between the body and the environment that feels concussive, there is contact that penetrates (John's stabbing pain), constricts (Rachel's viselike sinus headaches), or heats up (Mr. H's burning pain). We may also experience combinations of these (Price's white-hot branding iron, or the hot barbed wire encircling the spine of another patient at the pain clinic). Such combinations might evoke a certain smell (of burning matter) and taste (the metallic taste of iron). Here too we can learn from writers and patients. By emphasizing, even exaggerating, the physicality of an agent, they are able to communicate their pain more effectively. Instead of just stabbing, they may specify the type of knife or talk about multiple knives (Fanny Burney's mass of minute but sharp, forked poniards). Instead of just burning, they may talk about boiling hot water or a fire rapidly spreading down the leg (Mr. H). Such images make these experiences more meaningful to patients and, ideally, also to doctors, who must see and believe pain before they can treat it.

At the same time, we must keep the metaphor simple and straightforward. The agent capable of producing such horrific damage to the body must be seen as the direct cause of pain. That is why London points unambiguously to the White Silence, not an aging tree or human fallibility, as responsible for the suffering of his characters:

The cold of space smote the unprotected tip of the planet, and he, being on that unprotected tip, received the full force of the blow.

This representation is not entirely accurate, as London must have known. In the case of hypothermia, for example, the body itself is actually responsible for much of the pain. It responds to the cold by altering the normal pattern of circulation, cutting off blood supply to the periphery (hands, feet, nose, ears) and diverting it (and the warmth it carries) to vital organs of the interior (heart and lungs). In this way, the body intentionally sacrifices its expendable parts, causing them to undergo frostbite and necrosis. Yet when we try to convey the experience, we must be careful not to complicate the picture by saying that the cold and the body combined forces to destroy our fingers and ears. Instead, it is the cold alone—it "smites." Similarly, the wind in "The House of Mapui" is imagined as making it impossible for a person to breathe, even though his body (through the diffuse muscle contraction that prevents the lungs from fully expanding) bears some of the blame:

> The wind strangled him. He could not face it and breathe, for it rushed in through his mouth and nostrils, distending his lungs like bladders. At such moments it seemed to him that his body was being packed and swollen with solid earth. Only by pressing his lips to the trunk of the tree could he breathe.

This causal complexity extends to many common agents of disease and pain: viruses, bacteria, even cancer. The body produces fever and malaise, not the influenza virus. The itch from a mosquito bite is caused by mast cells in our skin (and the molecules they release) as much as the bite itself. The far-reaching destruction and pain in tuberculosis patients is caused more by the body's overzealous immune response to the organism than by the organism itself. And the list goes on.

To represent such experiences, our best bet is a simple, direct picture: the wind is strangling me; the flu is burning me up; tuberculosis is ravaging my lungs. We do this because the experiences are vague and abstract to begin with and we don't want to add to that vagueness. For the same reason, we typically prefer an external agent (the wind, the cold, or the mosquito) to an internal one (the muscles of the chest wall, the circulatory system, or mast cells in the skin), which is much less knowable for most people.

PAIN AS INTENTIONAL

If literary agency can be drawn out progressively—the more elaborate the metaphor, the more closely it approximates the experience of pain—then a possible endpoint might occur when an agent is invested with a destructive will. Initially the environment as agent was objectified, given a capital letter, and dissociated from its prospective victims ("The White Silence"). Next, the objectified environment became animated as it began to move against the sufferer ("The First Snowfall," "Lost on the Steppe"), and then when it acquired the capacity to announce its own threat ("The Open Boat"). Later its material or bodily presence was emphasized ("The Heathen," "The House of Mapui"). Last, the environment can be pictured as moving its "body" in purposeful ways.

What gradually emerges at the end of this sequence is ourselves, human beings with forms and actions. It is as if the person in pain, or the author on his behalf, responds like God by creating an agent in his own image. Thus the agent re-presents the felt experience of pain in external form (verbal and visible) at the same time as it re-presents the human body (or certain of its characteristics) around which the experience takes place; the agent is made up of the same material it will harm.

The emergence of the human body in representations of pain should come as no surprise. As Elaine Scarry reminds us, the projection of our "aliveness" onto nonsentient objects, be it the wind or the ocean or even a story about a person in pain, is a central motif in all acts of creation, one that shows up over and over again along the historic arc of civilization.

The habit of poets and ancient dreamers to project their own aliveness onto nonalive things itself suggests that *it is* the basic work of creation to bring about this very projection of aliveness; in other words, while the poet pretends or wishes that the inert external world had his or her own capacity for sentient awareness, civilization works to make this so. What in the poet is recognizable as a fiction is in civilization unrecognizable because it has come true.

We can see the consequences of the creative act in literature when an author and reader join together to breathe life into a fictional character, a being made up entirely of letters and words on a piece of paper. We can also see them in the double transformation of the environment in the particular works we have been discussing, when the words first become animated and then assume a human form.

The motivation behind these "projections of aliveness" is an ongoing attempt to understand ourselves and the world around us. Earlier I alluded to the work of Mark Johnson, who elegantly demonstrates that even the most abstract concepts are grounded in our physical (or bodily) interactions with the environment. Our basic physical experiences of balance—trying to stand up as a baby, for example, and learning how to ride a bicycle—ultimately give rise (through the imagination and metaphor) to our understanding of concepts like argument, justice, and mathematics. Now, pain on first blush may appear to be as basic a physical experience as balance. Yet because of its underlying structure (or, more accurately, *lack* of structure), pain seems much more elusive, much more like our abstract concepts. That is why a sufferer, trying to make his experience intelligible, will reduce its complexity by grounding it in even more basic and knowable experiences. Like the Romantic poets, who personified the natural world around them, we human beings make sense of complicated phenomena (whether pain or beauty or justice) in human terms— terms, observe Johnson and George Lakoff in *Metaphors We Live By*, "that we can understand on the basis of our own motivations, goals, actions, and characteristics."

A humanlike agent might not only possess mass but be capable of wielding its mass. Just like a person with a complex neuromuscular system, it should be able to exert force in a highly specific manner, like the wind in a poem by James Stephens:

> The wind stood up and gave a shout
> He whistled on his fingers, and
>
> Kicked the withered leaves about
> And thumped the branches with his hand
>
> And said he'll kill, and kill, and kill:
> And so he will! And so he will?

Stephens's wind reminds us of Hardy's wind, which was equally nimble as it trampled, climbed, sprang, and shrieked. More important, it too was an agent of destruction, capable of inflicting pain and killing like a human being, for this is precisely what the wind did to Grace's lover, Giles, who faced its wrath in his unprotected and weakened state.

In the South Pacific hurricane depicted in Jack London's "The Heathen," the ocean effortlessly flings "human fruit" off coconut trees and decimates an enormous ship. It behaves with such intent and agility, in fact, that it becomes difficult to call it an ocean, a supposedly senseless body of water:

> The sea rose. It jumped, it leaped, it soared straight toward the clouds. . . . The seas sprang from every point of the compass . . . They were hollow, maniacal seas. . . . They were not seas at all.

Description in the negative soon yields to a more positive formulation as the sea is pictured as first an inebriated and later a psychotic person:

> They were splashes, monstrous splashes. . . . They were drunken. They fell anywhere, anyhow. They jostled one another; they col-

lided. They rushed together and collapsed upon one another. . . .
It was no ocean that any man ever dreamed of, that hurricane center. . . . It was anarchy. It was a hell-pit of sea-water gone mad.

In a similar way, Tolstoy's wind "peevishly tosses" his character's col-
lar and then "insultingly slaps him."

By viewing pain in terms not just of agency but more specifically
of human agency, these writers continue to make the experiences of
their characters more meaningful. The man in London's hurricane
can barely breathe. He feels as if he's being strangled. But if the
feeling is to make sense to the man and to the reader of the story,
the event must be radically transformed. The wind, an inanimate
entity that strikes arbitrarily, cannot *literally* strangle him (just as it
cannot *literally* slap Tolstoy's character). So it must be remade to
strangle metaphorically, to be able to act with the dexterity and
power of a human being.

This same need to make sense of pain is no less pervasive in the
clinic and hospital. Patients can't suffer without wanting to know
why, without searching for a cause. They are hardly satisfied when
doctors tell them that there is no reason they developed diabetes or
cancer, that such diseases just happen. Nor does pointing to genetics
or random mutations help. Someone or something has to be held
responsible, either the patient himself (for eating the wrong food or
living the wrong life) or someone else who has it in for him (God, the
previous doctor, an uncaring spouse, or any other imagined scape-
goat). This is why Reynolds Price doesn't stay long with the image of
his spinal cord tumor as an inert branding iron; a lethal eel that feeds
its own destructive needs at Price's expense makes more sense. It is
why James Gillray, the British caricaturist, represents the pain he
suffers from gout as a fire-snorting devil, digging its fangs malevo-
lently into his swollen foot. And it is why the patient with a growing
mass in the lungs that blocks his airway imagines that someone is
strangling him. Cancer has become a someone, not just a thing, that
is actively against him—an enemy intent on destroying him.

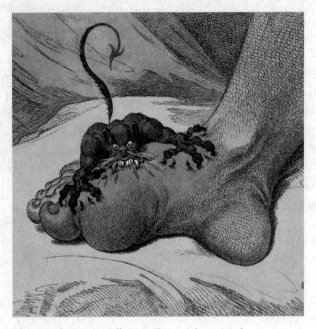

The Gout by James Gillray. *Wellcome Library, London.*

But is this really metaphorical progress? Isn't there something troubling, almost paranoid, about these last incarnations of agency, when pain or cancer is transformed into an evil person?

Perhaps we have reached a tipping point of sorts, for while the agency metaphor seems to be narrowing in on the phenomenology of pain, it is also moving in the opposite direction. The metaphor turns ambiguous. True, it seems to have captured the aversiveness of pain—we really feel as if there is an enemy bent on destroying us. But at a certain point it also seems to veer beyond our feelings, focusing more on what caused them (and the metaphorical vehicle used to convey them). The narrative of pain becomes instead the narrative of agency. And finding a human agent is just another attempt to zero in on the "Why?" of pain.

A weapon is no longer good enough. Now we need to find the party responsible for using it—for pulling the trigger, so to speak.

John's pain is stabbing; if that's the case, there must be a knife; but a knife doesn't stab on its own; so there must be person wielding the knife. Or Mr. H's burning pain that feels like his leg is on fire—well, then, who started the fire? The problem is that there is no end to this line of questioning. We might next ask how someone started the fire and why.

This potential instability is precisely what Susan Sontag rails against in her critique of metaphor in illness. When we shift our focus to the secondary subjects or vehicles of metaphor (agents and war), we lose sight of the primary subjects. We lose sight of the *pain* and *illness* that brought us to metaphor in the first place. In the case of the military metaphor, for example, doctors (like Shaw's farcical physician or the oncologists in Margaret Edson's play *Wit*) become more concerned with stimulating phagocytes and destroying cancer than with making the patient well (or at least more comfortable as she dies). It also leads to a host of other harmful and often ridiculous notions—that God, for example, or patients themselves (because they are repressed or extroverted, religious or atheistic), are ultimately responsible for their suffering. And if we can't find a reason in this world, then perhaps we'll find one in the next one. "I shall know why," writes Emily Dickinson:

> when time is over—
> And I have ceased to wonder why—
> Christ will explain each separate anguish
> In the fair schoolroom of the sky—
>
> He will tell me what "Peter" promised—
> And I—for wonder at his woe—
> I shall forget the drop of Anguish
> That scalds me now—that scalds me now!

These considerations force us to modify our initial claim, that the progressive elaboration of agency continues to shed light on the experience of pain. For in these last formulations, when an agent materializes first into a person and then into God, we have moved a great distance away from the body in pain and our understanding of it. Therefore, we must revise our strictly positive account of metaphor's epistemological value. While the language of agency is no doubt extremely helpful for people in pain, it also has a problematic side. People who suffer naturally want to know why. They grasp for explanations, for causes, which are partially fulfilled through metaphor. But what remains unanswered or left out becomes a new source of concern, necessitating further exploration. The search for knowledge is like an infinite regress, with a sufferer desiring to know and constantly being thwarted. We might have sensed this problem in the almost endless enumeration of weight in London's stories and in the reports of cardiac patients—not sand but mud, not a car but a freight train; and even these descriptions are not quite right.

Yet what would be a satisfying conclusion to the search? Can there even be a conclusion? Earlier it was suggested that if pain is by its nature intentionless, it can be imaginatively reconceived as being intentional. Hence we are drawn to the metaphor of agency. However, when pain (and illness) are considered in increasingly militaristic terms, the fact that war is in some sense a *purposive* activity cannot fail to underscore by contrast the often *purposelessness* of pain. This is especially true in cases of chronic pain where there is no tissue damage, no ongoing threat to the sufferer, and where pain, according to Reynolds Price, "signifies nothing." What drops out of the metaphor is precisely this significance, which, in the case of war, makes the horrific destruction at least somewhat intelligible. Pain has the impact and insistence of purposive action but no seeming end point or goal.

Metaphor promises us a solution to the linguistic and conceptual crises we face. It offers an antidote to the elusiveness and blankness of experiences like pain. Grounded in a desire for presence, metaphor expresses our craving, writes the philosopher Paul de Man, "to transform interior content into an outward thing." Sufferers, whether they live in literary texts or hospital wards, are deeply receptive to metaphor's power. While pain has no structure, form, or purpose, metaphors of pain *have* structure, form, and purpose; the experience becomes a story that has several characters and a plot with a beginning, a middle, and an end.

Problems arise, however, when we forget that the story is made up, when we cling to it as fact and continue to project the metaphor along absurd lines. It is at this point that rhetoric becomes transparently *fictional*; language turns in upon itself and becomes divorced from what it is supposed to represent, from the person in pain. Metaphor promises us control over experience by supplying it with meaning, and yet its representations are never absolute but are continuously being superseded by others in a self-perpetuating fashion. New representations give rise to new meanings, inevitably subverting the quest for a single, ultimate meaning.

Friedrich Nietzsche is even more vehement in his attack on rhetoric than de Man. For him, the distorting aspects of metaphor aren't limited to its fantastic elaborations. They are also present at its conception. Our tendency to attribute causality to certain phenomena is a perfect example. According to Nietzsche, we are not engaged in science (uncovering truth) but in art and metaphor (creating truth). In the case of pain, we feel awful and can't help but want to know why. We "find" a cause in the injured body, whether we see the damage or not. We experience pain *because* something must have struck and injured us; thus the agency metaphor is born. But that sequence is not necessarily accurate. In pain, there often is no "attack," and even when there is, it may not originate from the outside. We simply make things up as we go:

> We have learnt that all sensations which were ingenuously supposed to be conditioned by the outer world are, as a matter of fact, conditioned by the inner world: that the real action of the outer world

never takes place in a way that we can become conscious of. . . . That fragment of the outer world of which we become conscious, is born after the effect produced by the outer world has been recorded, and is subsequently interpreted as the "cause" of that effect.

In other words, we feel pain and *then* search for a cause. Our metaphorical imagination reorders the temporal sequence. Reflecting our desire to impose structure on events, it says, *No, that's not logical, that can't be how it is—first came the injury, then the pain.* Language, according to Nietzsche, blatantly misrepresents the facts.

The postmodern or deconstructionist view of language radically diverges from the more positive Wittgensteinian one discussed earlier. While Nietzsche believes that causality is imposed on phenomena from the outside (by language and mind), Wittgenstein might say that causality is an integral part of the experience of pain, which in turn enables language about pain to get under way. Taken absolutely, these viewpoints are as irreconcilable as the major controversies endlessly debated in philosophy (idealism versus realism) and biology (nature versus nurture). While I have been leaning in Wittgenstein's direction, there have been moments when the deconstructionist claims have been equally credible. Wittgenstein himself acknowledges that metaphors, or "pictures" as he calls them, can be misleading. Though we cannot do without them, we must recognize that a dogmatic adherence to a particular metaphor often leads to intellectual confusion: "A *picture* held us captive. And we could not get outside it, for it lay in our language and language seemed to repeat it to us inexorably."

Bearing this warning in mind—that we can "only safely use such language if we consciously remember the picture when we use it"—we cannot underestimate the positive and truly salutary role of the agency metaphor. Because of its elusiveness, pain resists language. The solution to this crisis, as Wittgenstein shows us, is to link the experience to public, observable phenomena, which is what happens when we learn the word "pain" and what is later reenacted in the language of agency. Pain is the feeling that something is moving against and injuring us, not just our bodies but our *selves* as a whole. Depending on the particular setting or type of pain, we feel certain parts of the narrative more intensely than others. At times it is the hostile trajectory of the agent that is emphasized—the agent as threat. At others, the impact or force of the agent on the body is most acutely felt and therefore emphasized. And finally there are times when we focus more intently on the "Why?" or the cause of pain.

The agency metaphor is flexible enough to accommodate these variations. Although it is not always apparent in the clinic and other ordinary language settings, we can easily appreciate its representational potential when the metaphor is used by skilled writers in literary settings. Some people will question the value or practicality of these literary versions of agency—whether they can possibly carry over into real-life situations. Should we start speaking like London and Tolstoy in front of our doctors? Say that our pain feels like Crane's growling waves coming at us? That our emphysema feels like London's wind, packing and swelling our airway with solid earth? That our lung cancer feels like someone is wrapping his hands around our trachea and strangling us?

Yes. Otherwise the experience will remain a private and unspoken one for us and will remain the same for other people too. The simple declaration "I am in pain" is often not enough to make the depths of our pain known and believable to doctors, family, and friends. If we want to communicate *effectively*, we must rely on the same strategies employed by our best writers. We must first objectify the experience by linking it with an agent and then emphasize whatever aspect of the experience is most pressing for us at the moment. If it is the sense of impending danger, we need to provide the agent with an appropriate form (London's White Silence, John's knife); we need to show that it is moving against us (Proulx's ocean rollers, Solzhen-itsyn's tanks, Maupassant's wind) and perhaps even announcing its threat (Tolstoy's howling wind, Crane's growling waves, the rumblings of Rachel's volcano). If it's the sense of collision or penetration, we can't just invoke an agent but must address what it is made of, how heavy it is, the sharpness of its edge, how hot or cold it is (London's wind packing millions of tons of sand, the cardiac patient's list of ever-bigger objects, Mr. H's fire-producing shingles). And if it's the desire to find a cause, we sometimes need to personify our agents (London's wind that strangles, Price's lethal eel hiding in his spinal cord, Gillray's gout-causing devil, Gilda Radner's war with cancer).

Only by doing so can we make pain more meaningful to ourselves and to others. Metaphor leads to knowledge and community.

8

The Mirror

And later, alone, the night grows inky, like my
thoughts, my thoughts . . . I turn to look out the
window: the gray buildings of my life,
the gray buildings.

—Lorrie Moore, "To Fill"

We left Hemingway's Harry several chapters ago, lying at the
foot of Mount Kilimanjaro with a gangrenous leg. Despite
having a well-meaning companion at his side, Harry feels isolated.
He is consumed by occurrences within his sick body that he cannot
share with others. No matter how hard he tries, his girlfriend
remains oblivious.

But Harry is also oblivious. Although he thinks the wound is serious, he is unsure and desperately wants more information. Is he
going to die? Is he in fact dying at that moment? While he sees his
leg growing more discolored, there is so much more that he cannot,
that remains inaccessible. Harry's sense that the wound is worse
than it looks is very much like the pain he feels—overwhelmingly
present but at the same time vague and indeterminate. He knows
yet does not know, and this uncertainty only adds to his suffering.

Harry turns to his girlfriend for help. *Can you feel the strange sensations I feel?* he asks, unable to fathom the possibility that what is
so urgent and real for him can be so distant and unreal for her. *Can
you help me find out how bad it is?* he asks, knowing full well that

she has no more insight than he has. Frustrated and alone, he confronts the crisis or epoché of pain.

But Harry doesn't resign himself to suffer silently, just like so many real-life patients who continue to talk and gesture even when convinced there is no point and like those who attempt to share their unimpartable experiences in the more structured forms of books and paintings. In the absence of human understanding, Harry must look elsewhere. He will find an alternative in an unlikely source—the vultures and hyena that assemble at the edges of the campsite. They will converse with him in more meaningful ways than his girlfriend. Because their powers of sight and smell exceed hers, they possess knowledge that she lacks. And when his girlfriend continues to insist that he will survive, Harry finally has had enough: "Don't be silly," he waves her away. "I'm dying now. Ask those bastards," he says, pointing to the vultures, which draw nearer every moment.

While the relationship that evolves with the scavengers is not sympathetic, it is a relationship nonetheless, one that involves a kind of dialogue. And when Harry attempts to articulate his suspicions, he pictures them in the form of a hyena:

> Just then it occurred to him that he was going to die. . . . It came with a rush; not as a rush of water nor of wind; but of a sudden evil-smelling emptiness and the odd thing was that the hyena slipped lightly along the edge of it.

Harry's sensations are elusive. He can't say what triggers them: a sudden pain, anxiety about the future, or the scent of decaying tissue. In order for him to make sense of things, he must look out into the world for meaning. There and only there can he find an appropriate form for his feelings:

> "I do [feel something strange]," he said. He had just felt death come by again . . . death had come and rested its head on the foot

of the cot and he could smell its breath. . . . [Death] can have a
wide snout like a hyena.

While the reader of Hemingway's story is more aware of what is
happening to Harry, the characters in the story that don't hear the
dialogue, even though they may be standing right next to Harry,
remain in the dark. It is only after Harry dies that the hyena speaks
to his girlfriend. Sensing the sufferer's last breath, the animal stops
"whimpering in the night" and begins to make a "strange, human,
almost crying sound." Harry's girlfriend, sleeping at the time, stirs
uneasily, and when the sound continues, she finally wakes up.

Hemingway's story employs a second type of metaphor: a metaphor
of projection. Like the language of agency, this metaphor links pain
to the external world. But instead of imagining objects that cause
pain, the sufferer imagines objects onto which he can project his
feelings and desires. The objects don't necessarily have to be other
human beings. They can be animals, like Hemingway's hyena and
vultures, which must be remade to communicate in terms humans
can understand. Or, as we will see, they can be inanimate entities,
like a tree, a piece of clothing, or Lorrie Moore's gray buildings,
which must be first imagined to experience pain and then made to
articulate it. Regardless of the object chosen, however, the motivation is the same: the person whose connection to the world has
been drastically severed must somehow create the world anew, one
that can understand him better and in which he can understand
himself better.

We will find that projection metaphors help the sufferer in three
fundamental ways. First, they can validate the experience both for
the person in pain and for an outside observer who might otherwise
be skeptical. Second, they can diminish the loneliness of pain by
making the world a more responsive place. And finally, there is a
reflexive quality in these metaphors that can not only enlarge the
world but also enlarge the self: the object that is remade to bear the

person's pain acts as a mirror in which the person can observe and understand what is happening to himself. Although we will discuss these goals separately, they are vitally integrated in the larger frame of what Nelson Goodman has called "worldmaking" and Elaine Scarry "creation." Language—in this case the metaphorical language of projection—leads to community and knowledge.

VALIDATING PAIN

Harry cannot understand the significance of the sensations in his leg. Though he believes he may be dying, he needs confirmation. Since his girlfriend can't provide it, he turns to the only other inhabitants of his rapidly shrinking world. The scavengers tell him what he wants to know, and for this reason he links them to his pain; they become what dying feels like to Harry.

Harry's need for confirmation is by no means unique. Illness, all illness, is rife with uncertainty. Patients are terrified when their bodies send out strange signals, when they develop symptoms they know aren't normal. What do the sensations mean? How serious are they? *What will happen to me?* Naturally, doctors, when available, can be consulted. But their answers may not be reassuring or entirely satisfying. Unfortunately, doctors aren't always the best communicators and don't often spend enough time with patients. Another problem is that most people overestimate the scientific basis of medicine. Even in the twenty-first century, the age of molecular biology and the Human Genome Project, most diseases remain mysterious, even common ones like hypertension and cancer. When patients ask why they got psoriasis or lupus and how it will play out for them, much of the time there really aren't any definite answers.

But it's not just knowledge in the form of diagnosis and prognosis that Harry and other patients urgently desire. They also want validation. The events occurring inside them are of overwhelming importance, even when not life-threatening. Patients can barely

focus on anything else. They desperately want someone to acknowledge what they are going through. I certainly did when I was a
patient. Though surrounded at all times by family and friends during my bone marrow transplant, I felt completely isolated. The
Great Wall of China had sprung up between us. Compassionate as
they were, my family couldn't feel or know how I felt. Like Harry's
girlfriend, they were standing on the far side of the wall. Nor could
I edge closer to them with language. At times the pain was so
unbearable it literally silenced me. And even when it subsided, I
could never find the right words.

Still, I was lucky. Things could have been worse. Instead of having so many sympathetic voices around, I might have had no one.
And as clueless as they were, my wife and parents firmly believed
that I was in great pain and tried as best as they could to comfort
me. That too isn't always a given. At times those on the far side of
pain's wall aren't sure. Just think of my patient Sandy, who woke in
the middle of the night to the incredulous look on her husband's
face; how could she possibly be in pain after three Percosets? There
are also times when skepticism can turn into disbelief, as in the case
of the sickle cell patient sent home without treatment from the
Kings County emergency room, or a friend of Rachel J's from the
pain clinic whose mysterious condition went ignored for years and
who ultimately resorted to self-mutilation to prove that she was suffering. Only when the patient produced a visual record of her pain—
the slash marks on her arm—did other people finally believe her.

These are not isolated incidents. We know that from medical studies showing that doctors routinely underprescribe analgesic medication to cancer and AIDS patients, despite their awareness that severe
pain can accompany these illnesses. How can this happen?

It happens because there is no definitive way to verify someone
else's pain, no foolproof, sophisticated test like an MRI or a PET
scan. In the end, all we have is the word of the sufferer, and we
must take that word on faith. And even if we believe that someone is
in pain, we can't always gauge the degree of pain or how much relief

is needed. To observe pain, Elaine Scarry has said, can be considered the primary model of what it is to have doubt: "For the person whose pain it is, it is 'effortlessly' grasped . . . while for the person outside the sufferer's body, what is 'effortless' is *not* grasping it (it is easy to remain wholly unaware of its existence . . .)."

Hemingway is keenly aware of the perceptual discrepancy between the person in pain and the observer of pain. He wants to minimize the discrepancy, to make Harry's pain so palpable that other people can't possibly ignore it. He does this by finding objects that can validate Harry's feelings. Because of their refined perceptions, the scavengers know that Harry is dying and are made to convey that knowledge to him. In doing so, they confirm not only his suspicions but also those of an outside observer. As Harry becomes more convinced, so does the reader of Hemingway's story. His girlfriend, however, who has known Harry for years but cannot read the metaphoric dialogue, continues to doubt.

A similar situation occurs in Maupassant's story "The First Snowfall," in which the husband dismisses his wife's suffering. It is not enough for her to say "I am cold and may soon become ill," just as it may not be enough for a cancer patient to say to a doctor, "I am still in pain and need more medicine." If we want others to believe us and take action, we need them to see the pain and appreciate its extent. Recognizing this need, Maupassant initially substantiates the cold's effect on the woman by objectifying it through metaphor, identifying a responsible agent (the cruel currents of air that incessantly buffet and threaten her). Then he uses another strategy, projecting his character's feelings onto an external object, which she can converse with:

> About four o'clock, the army of dark, flying creatures came and
> perched in the tall beeches at the left of the chateau, emitting
> deafening cries . . . they fluttered . . . seemed to be fighting,
> croaked, and made the gray branches move with their black wings.
> She gazed at them, each evening, with a pressure of the heart, so

deeply was she penetrated by the lugubrious melancholy of the night falling on desolate grounds.

The crows, whether they are part of the hostile environment or its victims, like the protagonist, *affect* the woman (from the Latin *affi-cere*); they make her as well as the reader aware of the imminent danger.

In this instance, projection works to represent the threat always present in the experience of pain, what we referred to in the last chapter as its signaling capacity. The crows—the objectification of the woman's feelings—act like biological warning bells; they alert the woman to danger so that she can take appropriate action.

But the critical nature of this capacity may be better appreciated when a threat doesn't register. Unlike Maupassant's woman, many of Jack London's characters are oblivious of the environment's destructive potential and die as a result. The tremendous cold of the Yukon makes no impression on the protagonist in one of London's most famous short stories, "To Build a Fire." He doesn't *see* the danger, which London assures the reader is unmistakably present. Nor does he *see* the warning signals that come from his body: the crackling of his spit in midair, the freezing of his facial hair, the muzzle of ice that binds his lips together. Finally, he ignores his only traveling companion, his dog, a creature who would be equally affected by the cold and who might alert the man. But what goes unrecognized by the man is very much in the minds of the readers of his story:

The animal was depressed by the tremendous cold. It knew that it was no time for traveling. Its instinct told it a truer tale than was told to the man by the man's judgment. . . . The dog did not know anything about thermometers. Possibly in its brain there was no sharp consciousness of a condition of very cold such as was in the man's brain. But the brute had its instinct. It experienced a vague but menacing apprehension that subdued it and made it slink along at the man's heels, and that made it question eagerly every unwanted movement of the man as if expecting him to go into camp or to seek shelter somewhere and build a fire.

What becomes increasingly apparent to the person in pain, to the author who attempts to convey pain, and perhaps most of all to the reader of a story about pain is the sheer invisibility of the experience. The quality of pain, its locus, its verifiability—all lack the density that might enable a sufferer, author, and reader to grasp it. And as so many of London's stories make clear, the inability to grasp it often has life-threatening consequences. At the same time, the stories suggest ways to counteract pain's elusiveness. While London's man is "quick and alert," he has little imagination. If we want to be able to represent pain, to make it mean something, we have to use our imagination and objectify the experience through metaphor.

Remember young Stephen Dedalus, who experiences fever and chills? Lacking the skills of language, Stephen imagines a faucet in his body alternately running hot and cold water. Harry, who is older, is dying and cannot convey his sensations to his companion. The scavengers, though, are receptive. Harry's pain becomes the hyena with its foul-smelling snout. Maupassant's woman's pain, the crows that croak in the night. These objects are not the equivalent of experience, just as words are not. But as signs, as representations of internal phenomena, they stand in for experience, and because they stand in the external world, visible and palpable, they can be shared with other people. As such, they can help validate a person's pain.

Nor do the benefits of being able to represent pain end here. Implicit in the creation of a sign, whereby something signified (pain) becomes linked to a signifier (object), is its functionality. The sign is a signal that calls for a response, that requires what the philosopher C. S. Peirce once called an "interpretant"; it creates meaning, inasmuch as one can act on that meaning. Thus Stephen will go to the infirmary. Maupassant's woman will ask for a furnace. And though Harry will die, the objectification of his experience in the form of a hyena gives him something palpable to grab on to during his last moments, like the comfort Nietzsche gets from giving his pain a name:

I have given a name to my pain and call it "dog"; it is just as faithful, just as obtrusive and shameless . . . and I can scold it and vent
my bad mood on it, as others do with their dogs.

London's man without imagination, in contrast, while aware of the
freezing cold, is oblivious of its significance for him. And because he
has not recognized the threat, because he has not read its signs
accurately, he will continue to suffer instead of heeding the advice
of his dog and finding shelter that might save his life.

CREATING A RESPONSIVE WORLD

Throughout this book our focus has shifted back and forth between
the felt experience of pain and verbal representations of that experience. In the stories and clinical cases just discussed, for example,
metaphors of projection are used to validate pain. That such metaphors are necessary leads us back to the experience itself, especially
to a person's feeling that his pain may not be believed.

A second goal of projection metaphors is to create a more
responsive world. By linking their experience to the hyena and the
crows, Harry and Maupassant's woman identify objects that speak
to them and to whom they in turn may respond. Unable to communicate with their human companions, they will converse with
anybody or anything that will listen to them, and it is now the dialogue rather than the object itself that is important to the sufferer.
To appreciate why this is so, we need to revisit the felt experience
of pain, and in particular its "element of blank," which the metaphor is called upon to fill.

Pain, we have said, radically transforms our perspective, from the
normal outward-facing one to the abnormal and distressing inward-
facing one. As the body enlarges in significance, the world beyond
contracts in inverse proportion: "A bandage hides the place where
each is living." Life is no longer outside us, in our jobs and relationships and pleasurable pursuits. It is inside us, in the head that throbs

and the hand that hurts every time we try to move it. That's what really matters at the moment. Moreover, the body becomes progressively fragmented as one of its parts, the locus of pain, assumes precedence over the whole: "For who when healthy can become a foot?" Since I can focus only on my head or my hand, the rest of me suddenly becomes superfluous. In fact, that's all I am right now—a throbbing head, a hurting hand.

Yet these feelings of progressive inwardness and fragmentation are a dead end. As a foot or a hand, I can no longer relate to other people, nor can they relate to me—so why bother trying? They also don't take into account the equally real (though less conspicuous) impulse that pushes us in the opposite direction, away from the self and toward the world, that urges us to find meaning and convey it: I don't want to be a foot or live like a mollusk and will do everything in my power to escape and return to family and friends. For this reason, we should revise our notion of lived existence, whether in health or in illness. As Maurice Merleau-Ponty suggests, being is never directed exclusively in one direction or another but is rather a dialectic that thrusts us inward at one moment and outward the next.

The short stories we have been discussing effectively capture this dialectic. The characters who come to experience pain are literally situated at the outermost boundaries of civilization. With few or no companions, they are alone in the vast, desolate expanse of the Yukon, the Caucasus, or the Atlantic Ocean. The more symbolic distance separating a patient in the hospital from the rest of the world—the Great Wall that sprang up between me and my family, or Bauby's diving bell, which sends him down into the ocean depths—becomes for them an actual one. We might say that the extremity of these situations represents the central conflict in the stories, as it always does in the real-life dramas of the ill.

Yet while they emphasize the isolation of a person in pain, the stories equally emphasize the opposite extreme, the need to find community. They are essentially Merleau-Ponty's thought experiment (the transcendental reduction or epoché) in the form of narrative.

Paradoxically, it is by bracketing the world, by putting it "out of play," that we ultimately realize that it is unbracketable and that we begin to appreciate the dialectic between human being and world where meaning is generated: "Man is in the world and only in the world does he know himself." As the characters in these stories reach for meaning through metaphor, they engage in worldmaking; they remake their unresponsive surroundings to be responsive. In this way the "intentional threads" that link them to the world can be seen *as they emerge* from the void, which is why we said that pain, and stories of pain, provide us with an extraordinary opportunity to witness the way language and meaning come into being.

In Harry's remaking, the hyena is credited with a special sensitivity to what is happening inside his body. In addition, it is able to communicate this knowledge to him. Finally, it becomes the objectified form of what dying feels like. In Maupassant's woman's remaking, the crows are made to perceive the danger posed by the cold; they are able to convey this knowledge to her (by affecting her); and finally they become the objectification of an inner experience, the woman's anxiety. One only wishes that London's man might have been better at worldmaking, for if the environment were credited with expressivity (as it was for London's readers), if the warning signs from his body and that of his dog had actually registered, perhaps he might have averted disaster.

Philosophers like Maurice Merleau-Ponty reject the isolating philosophies derived from Descartes' *cogito*—I think, therefore I am—because they run counter to the fundamentally social nature of lived existence. The privileging of the thinking self inevitably leads to alienation; it separates the mind from the body and the individual from other people. By viewing existence dialectically, however—by thinking in terms of a person as an embodied consciousness and of an ongoing dialogue between person and world—the strict ontological divisions between these entities diminish in importance. But it's not so much that Merleau-Ponty cares whether the tree in the forest *exists* independently of our seeing. What is more critical for him is that the unseen tree *has no meaning* or significance independent of our seeing. Like any object in the world, the tree is not a tree *in-itself* but a tree *for-us*; its meaning emerges in the way we see, talk about, and use the tree in our everyday lives: "The object 'speaks' and is significant in our activity with it."

A perfect place to witness the dialogue between subjects and objects is in our habits, our daily interactions with things like a computer keyboard or a cane. Here the connection between person and thing becomes so intense that it is often difficult to identify where one surface ends and the other begins. In learning to walk with a cane, suggests Merleau-Ponty, we alter our entire "corporeal schema." The body (or, more precisely, the hand that grips the cane) is extended by several feet; we begin to feel the pavement as it makes contact with the tip of the cane as if, on the one hand, we are actually touching the pavement, or, on the other hand, the cane has come to acquire tactile perception:

> To get used to a hat, a car, or a stick is to be transplanted into them or conversely, to incorporate them into the bulk of our own body. Habit expresses the power of dilating our being-in-the-world, or changing our existence by appropriating fresh instruments.

In a sense, we merge with the object—it takes on a little of us and we take on a little of it, a merging that also opens up the lines of communication. We can hear the resulting dialogue more clearly perhaps when we stub our toe and then curse the ground, as if the ground (onto which we project human attributes) can be culpable and hear our disapproval; or when we feel the side of our car collide with another vehicle, as if it were our own body that suffers the impact. As Merleau-Ponty recognized, we converse with the world to make sense of it and create meaning in our lives.

What distinguishes this common yet thoroughly metaphorical activity in the setting of illness and pain is the urgency with which we draw on it. These are crisis situations that threaten to erase the world and everything in it. We desperately want to escape the soli-

tude and find our way back. Being able to express how we feel and
having someone listen would be a step in the right direction. But
there aren't always other people around. And even when there are,
they may not be as receptive as we might wish: doctors who barely
glance at us; friends who may not believe us; family members who
can't bear to witness the uglier sides of illness or simply prefer not to
be bothered by our endless complaints.

Not surprisingly, patients are constantly looking for fellow sufferers on their side of the Great Wall. Sandy, my patient with rheumatoid arthritis, finds comfort in talking to her mother, who has the
same illness and has gone through just about everything she has:
years of suffering and disability, a variety of different medications
and doctors, bilateral knee and hip replacements. Even when conversation becomes stilted, which happens between parents and children, Sandy always has a sympathetic ear that she can count on.

Most others will need to enlarge their "families" by adopting
patients with similar diagnoses. Despite starting off as complete
strangers, these new family members can understand what the
healthy and pain-free can never understand. They, too, will probably
want to talk and listen. Alphonse Daudet calls the fellow sufferers
he meets at Lamalou, the sanatorium in France where he is treated
for syphilis, his "doppelgangers in pain":

> My doppelganger. The fellow whose illness most closely resembles
> your own. How you love him, and how you make him tell you every-
> thing! I've got two such, an Italian painter and a member of the
> Court of Appeal. Between them, these two comprise my suffering.

Nowadays it's even easier to find sympathetic voices. Patients can
belong to support groups or search for doppelgangers on the World
Wide Web, in Internet chat rooms and on blogs.

Still, there will be times when no one is around and when all we
have left is our imagination. Then we must rely, like the fictional
characters we have considered, on metaphor to remake our worlds.
If our spouses or doctors won't listen to us, then we must find others

who will, like the hyena and the crows. Even things that can't literally experience pain can be remade to listen: a character in a book or
a movie, for example, with whom we identify; a song that "knows"
exactly how we feel, like the Carly Simon song we think is about us;
or the natural world when it miraculously mirrors our internal one—
the gloomy sky that shares our sadness, the inky sky that shares our
madness (as in this chapter's epigraph).

In the previous chapter we saw that nature (the wind and waves)
could be given a voice to show that it was acting on the sufferer like
an agent. Now, in the language of projection, nature will speak to us
to show that it experiences pain just as we do. In this way, the metaphor not only makes our interior experience visible but also brings
us the companionship we desperately need.

Tolstoy ascribes such a voice to nature in "Master and Man." The
story centers on the journey of Vasili, a bourgeois merchant who
hopes to add more land to his estate, and Nikita, his faithful servant, whom he berates at every turn. During the journey, the travelers find themselves increasingly isolated in a frozen Russian
wilderness that threatens their existence. As a result, the narrative
progresses like the narrative of pain, in effecting an epoché. As the
two men turn inward, the world, which previously provided comfort, gradually begins to recede, until there is nothing left to see,
hear, and feel but their bodies in pain:

> The road could hardly be seen. . . . For a few moments they heard
> the panting of the tired little horse and the drunken shouting of the
> peasants. Then the panting and the shouts died away, and around
> them nothing could be heard but the whistling of the wind in their
> ears. . . . In spite of his efforts nothing could be heard but the wind
> whistling between the shafts, the flapping of the kerchief, and the
> snow pelting against the frame of the sledge.

At the same time, the two men become separated. They can't hear
each other speak because their voices are mangled by the wind.

But despite this seemingly absolute epoché, Vasili refuses to be alone. He searches for others in the white waste with whom he can talk and sort things out. First he notices a tall oak tree "which had a few dry leaves still dangling on it." Next he encounters stalks of wormwood "sticking up through the snow and swaying in the wind." Later on he sees the willow trees fluttering in the breeze and making "melancholy sounds." Finally, on three separate occasions, the willows begin to "moan sadly."

The trees are speaking to Vasili. They are speaking to him about himself. The snow pressing down upon their branches is likewise pressing down upon his limbs. The wind is pounding against both defenseless bodies. What does it all mean?

> Stalks of wormwood, sticking up through the snow . . . and desperately tossing about under the pressure of the wind which beat it all to one side and whistled through it. The sight of that wormwood tormented by the pitiless wind made Vasili Andreevich shudder, he knew not why.

The "conversation" gradually helps Vasili clarify his experience. He has made a grave error, not just in this particular instance but throughout his entire life. He has treated others—his wife, his son, his servant, the trees he buys and sells, and even his God—as objects that exist only to enhance his wealth. Now, however, in a King Lear–like moment, when the agonizing cold has penetrated his body and no one is present to hear his pain, he turns to the trees for sympathy. They must hurt as he does, and it is awful to see someone in pain:

> He thought of the wormwood tossed by the wind, which he had twice ridden past, and he was seized with such terror that he did not believe in the reality of what was happening to him. . . . It was real snow that lashed his face and chilled his right hand from which he had lost the glove, and this was a real desert in which he

was now left alone like that wormwood, awaiting an inevitable, speedy, and meaningless death.

The pain Vasili experiences is within him and all-consuming. In his desperation, he literally attempts to flee from it. But when at last he turns to the trees and pictures them feeling the way he feels, he begins to understand. The unexpected revelation of suffering is so powerful that it motivates Vasili to make the ultimate selfless act before he dies.

He is no longer fearful when he comes upon the "something" that turns out to be the half-dead body of Nikita. Without hesitation, Vasili proceeds to cover the body of his servant—the same servant to whom he tried to sell a bad horse, at whom he sneered for being uneducated and poorly dressed, and whose life he belittled as meaningless—with his own body. Acting selflessly, he keeps Nikita's body warm while his own body freezes.

By attributing a voice to the trees, Vasili repopulates his increasingly barren world with responsive beings. He acts, the literary critic Jonathan Culler might say, like the Romantic poets, who routinely addressed the ocean and clouds and other inanimate objects around them in order to find companionship:

> The object is treated as a subject, an I which implies a certain type of you in its turn. One who successfully invokes nature is one to whom nature might, in its turn, speak. He makes himself poet, visionary.

All artists work to make things speak which ordinarily don't—letters or dabs of paint on a piece of paper or the things that those letters and paint represent (Tolstoy's trees, Munch's figure). They do this with an ulterior motive: to make themselves speak, to express their innermost feelings. This is a task that is never easy, as the philosopher Susanne Langer observes, and as any person who experiences pain knows all too well:

It may seem strange that the most immediate experiences in our lives should be the least recognized, but there is a reason for this apparent paradox, and the reason is precisely their immediacy. They pass unrecorded because they are known without any symbolic mediation, and therefore without conceptual form. We usually have no objectifying images of such experiences to recall and recognize, and we do not often try to convey them in more detail than would be likely to elicit sympathy from other people.

Because felt, inner activity lacks form, like thought without language, it passes largely unknown to those who live it. The artist, however, attempts to articulate "the movement of emotive and perceptive processes" by projecting them onto "extraorganic structures," by formulating them in symbols and images. Once created, the symbol—an abstraction of the phenomenal content of feeling—is fixed in the artist's medium and presented to a reader (or viewer or listener).

Vasili's metaphor of the trees in pain, like the need of many real patients to seek out fellow sufferers and to project their feelings onto songs and gloomy skies, provides form for his experience. Isolated, suffering, and voiceless, Vasili responds by remaking the world and filling it with objects that can hear him, sympathize with him, and speak to him of himself. In this way he begins the healing process. The metaphor works like (and in the absence of) medicine; it has the power to alleviate pain.

UNDERSTANDING OUR PAIN

When we look out at the world, we see ourselves. In this way, we are truly and irreducibly in the world, bringing us to the third goal of projection metaphors, which underlies and serves as the overriding intention of the other two. By substantiating the experience of pain in an object, by making that object responsive, a person is at the same time engaged in the process of constituting himself. As

Merleau-Ponty says, the world does not merely speak but speaks to us about our *selves*. The bridging of the ontological division between a person (subject) and the world (object) inevitably leads to a narrowing in the epistemological domain. People don't know themselves and other people and things in isolation. We know ourselves and the world through our ongoing dialogue with it. Man is not only *in* the world, he *knows* himself in the world.

In the thick of grief, the poet Mark Doty tells us in his memoir, *Heaven's Coast*, that he inhabits a dark, empty space "like the socket of a pulled tooth." His lover of twelve years has just died of AIDS. As he walks along the beach on Cape Cod, he spots a seal stranded on a low rise of sand ahead of him. The seal appears exhausted and distressed. Did an especially high tide bring it there? he wonders. Or did the seal purposely pull itself out of the water to rest? As he moves closer, Doty observes that the seal's face is suffused with "helplessness and desolation." Although the seal bears no visible wound, it is clearly in pain, a deeper kind of pain, and this cuts Doty to the core. He is looking into the mirror and seeing himself—himself in a deep, lonely pain. The dark, empty space of grief is now replaced with the vivid face of the seal in front of him. Doty can see it and reflect on it and in doing so reflect on himself.

For Paul D, a character in Toni Morrison's *Beloved*, the catalyst for self-knowledge is a rooster on the plantation where he is enslaved. He first identifies with the bird when its egg won't hatch and he has to help the deformed creature with crooked legs out of the shell. Just like him, it is a "throw-away" thing, and Paul D is determined to watch over it.

But the rooster evolves over time, altering the self-portrait it helps Paul D create. After a failed escape, the slave is brutally shackled and a horse's bit is placed in his mouth. The pain of the iron yanking back the lips and slamming down on the tongue is excruciating. Yet that wasn't what hurt most, he explains to Sethe years later. It was the rooster looking at him and smiling. No longer an outcast, the rooster had become Mister, boss of the roosters, perched on his bathtub throne and assessing Paul D with a hateful, bloody gaze. It was at that moment that Paul D recognized what he had become, and the pain of this recognition proved too much for him to bear. *I swear*, he tells Sethe, *Mister smiled*:

> When I saw Mister, I knew it was me too. Not just them, me too. One crazy, one sold, one missing, one burnt and me licking iron with my hands crossed behind me. The last of the Sweet Home Men.
>
> Mister, he looked so . . . free. Better than me. Stronger, tougher. Son a bitch couldn't even get out the shell by hisself but he was still king and I was . . .
>
> Mister was allowed to be and stay what he was. But I wasn't allowed to be and stay what I was. Even if you cooked him, you'd be cooking a rooster named Mister. But wasn't no way I'd ever be Paul D again, living or dead. Schoolteacher changed me. I was something else and that something was less than a chicken sitting in the sun on a tub.

When he looked into the metaphorical mirror on that fateful day, Paul D realized that his life as a human being had ended, just as it had for his fellow slaves. From then on he would bury every last trace of feeling—pain and pleasure—in the tobacco tin in his chest "where a red heart used to be. Its lid rusted shut."

Mark Doty's and Toni Morrison's literary conceits, where a poet and a character in a novel see themselves in a seal and in a rooster, are projection metaphors. But this kind of metaphor isn't used only by artists. All of us are constantly looking for and finding ourselves in other people and things, especially when we are ill and in pain. Patients with similar conditions can validate our experiences and provide a sympathetic ear. They can also help us understand ourselves.

After her stroke, Julia Fox Garrison tells us in her memoir, *Don't Leave Me This Way*, she eagerly sought out information about other patients on her hospital ward—how they were feeling, how they were doing. She did this not so much because she cared about them but because she cared about *herself*. What could they tell her about how she was feeling and doing?

> Is there anybody like me here? Is there anybody who is 37 years old who has a 3-year-old child? I would like to know if there is anyone who mirrors me here, anyone I can identify with.

Garrison is terrified of what the stroke has done to her, so she looks for doppelgangers that might help orient her to her strange, new, paralyzed self.

Toward the end of his life, Alphonse Daudet could no longer walk steadily. The ataxia caused by syphilitic damage to his cerebellum resulted in a clumsy, halting gait. But the only way for him to see what he looked like was to observe himself in a mirror or, better yet, to observe another patient in the hospital who had the same problem:

> I see him in my mind's eye, putting one foot down carefully before the other, but still tottery: as if walking on ice. Sad.

No doubt Daudet feels sad for his fellow sufferer. But he feels equally sad, if not more so, for himself and what has become of him.

We can also learn from people and things who are unlike us. Dr. Steven Hsi was in critical condition in the ICU when he began thinking about the sick baby in the bed next to him. The baby, worse off than he was, would die if she didn't get a heart transplant in the next few days. She was worse off in other ways too, Hsi decided, when his thoughts turned back to his own life:

> I was almost 42 years old and at least had the opportunity to have a childhood, to learn what it is like to fall in love, to marry, to have children and cherish them. I had been so fortunate. I had it pretty good actually. I was in no position to complain.

In this case, the seeing isn't a literal seeing, like Daudet observing himself in his doppelganger, but more the realization of how lucky Hsi has been relative to his unlucky neighbor.

Like fictional characters, patients find themselves in just about any object that happens to be on hand (or in the mind). Before his diagnosis, Daudet had a recurring dream that he was a boat whose keel kept scraping along the rocky sea bottom and causing him severe pain. The dreams became so vivid that he consulted a doctor to find out whether there might be something wrong with his own "keel." Indeed there was. Syphilis had eaten away at his spinal cord, the extensive damage triggering those intense paroxysms of pain he experienced during the night. Writing about how he felt later on, Daudet became the rotting ship of his dreams:

The ship is sinking. I'm going down, holed below the water-line. The flag's still nailed to the mast, but there's fire everywhere, even in the water. Beginning of the end. . . . The whole ship is falling apart.

Christian Wiman, in contrast, saw himself, like Tolstoy's Vasili, as a tree. The contemporary American poet was happily married and well on the way to a successful literary career when he was diagnosed with a rare blood disorder. Suddenly his life was placed on hold. He would get very sick, from the disease and from the treatment for it. He would be tested and might not survive, much like the apple sapling that grew next to his house and also battled a series of harsh, unexpected storms. "No remembering now," writes Wiman in his poem "After the Diagnosis":

When the apple sapling was blown
Almost out of the ground.
No telling how,
With all the other trees around,
It alone was struck . . .

He watched this tree survive
Wind ripping at his roof for nights
On end, heats and blights
That left little else alive.
No remembering now . . .
A day's changes mean all to him
And all days come down
To one clear pane
Through which he sees
Among all the other trees
This leaning, clenched, unyielding one
That seems cast
In the form of a blast
That would have killed it,
As if something at the heart of things,
And with the heart of things,
Had willed it.

Repeatedly beaten down like the apple sapling, Wiman prays that he too will remain standing when the storms finally pass.

Even abstract entities can be remade to mirror the felt experience of suffering. Soon after her stroke, Julia Fox Garrison was wheeled into the operating room on a gurney. That's when "Time," she writes in her memoir, "started to shudder," and kept shuddering until things became normal (relatively normal, that is) for her again.

Regardless of the kind of object we project our feelings onto (human, animal, insentient, or abstract) and regardless of the context (literary text, canvas, or the real world of the hospital), the motivation is the same. Unable to accept the elusive quality of pain, we want to pin it down and understand it. Only we can't do this by ourselves, for the source of pain, the human body, as intimate as we are with it, is difficult to know. Consider how little of what happens in our bodies we are consciously aware of, let alone able to perceive: the workings of the heart, lungs, liver, and other organs; the daily drama that goes on within the microscopic cells of the kidney or gastrointestinal tract; and, more remote still, life at the molecular level, where genes are constantly being turned on and off.

And it's not just the inside of the body that presents us with difficulties. I cannot, for example, observe my body's entire surface. Nor can I perceive it in full with my other senses. I need help. But what remains inaccessible for me may not be so for another person, who could examine my body as one might a sculpture in a museum and then tell me about it. Otherwise, I would need a mirror to see myself better. In both instances I am relying on an outside means to provide self-knowledge. Tolstoy's and Morrison's characters, like Mark Doty, Alphonse Daudet, Julia Fox Garrison, Steven Hsi, and Christian Wiman, are very much aware of their limitations in this regard. That is why they too turn to outside sources that can act as mirrors, enabling them to see themselves.

At the turn of nineteenth-century France, a revolution occurred in the field of medicine. As the theorist and historian Michel Foucault explains in *The Birth of the Clinic*, the revolution was motivated by the same inaccessibility of the human body that motivates fictional and actual sufferers to use projection metaphors. Physicians then were no better at diagnosing and treating patients than they had been centuries earlier. There was essentially a standstill in medical knowledge. Physicians could only speculate and theorize about the body, because they literally couldn't see into it and talk about what they saw. Without perception and language, there was no way to acquire empirical knowledge. For Bichat and other radical thinkers of the time, there was only one solution. They needed to exchange absence with presence:

At the beginning of the nineteenth century, doctors described what for centuries had remained below the threshold of the visible and the expressible, but this did not mean that, after over-indulging in speculation, they had begun to perceive once again. . . . It meant that the relation between the visible and the invisible—

which is necessary to all concrete knowledge—changed its structure, revealing through gaze and language what had previously been below and beyond their domain. A new alliance was forged between words and things, enabling one to see and to say.

While fictional and actual sufferers illuminate through metaphor, the French physicians illuminated more directly. They literally opened up the body (the dead body, that is, which was still relatively taboo at the time) and, by doing so systematically, created the field of pathological anatomy. Instead of imagining what was happening beneath the surface, they could now *see* for themselves—a *seeing* that for Foucault included all modes of perception. They also created the clinic (known today as the hospital), where sick people would go for evaluation and treatment. There physicians could observe many patients simultaneously and follow the course of their diseases over time. The net result of both projects was to situate disease in a world of constant visibility. At the moment that disease became accessible to the medical gaze, it could be talked about and known: "By saying what one sees, one integrates it spontaneously into knowledge."

As so many contemporary thinkers like Foucault have recognized, we simply can't get very far by ourselves. Knowledge depends on the presence of others: other people, like doctors and patients; and other things, like dead bodies, deformed roosters, and suffering trees. That holds true for knowledge about the world (medicine) as it does for knowledge about the self (our own bodies). Ordinarily our focus is more outward than inward. We hardly notice or give much thought to our bodies when healthy. We pass by them in silence, suggests Jean-Paul Sartre. But that is not the case when we are ill and in pain. Then the inside world is the only thing that matters. Then we must see and know what is happening there. Only we can't do this from our perspective alone. We need another perspective. Paradoxically, we can see the inside only from the outside, from the other's point of view. It appears to us, writes Sartre, "that the Other accomplishes for us a function of which we are incapable and which nevertheless is incumbent on us: *to see ourselves as we are.*"

By linking ourselves (who can't be very objective) with others (who can be more so), we gain access to ourselves. We can observe and discuss, and thereby know, what was previously unintelligible.

MIRROR NEURONS: A BIOLOGICAL BASIS FOR PROJECTION

Twenty years ago, researchers in the small Italian city of Parma made a fascinating discovery. Certain neurons in the brains of monkeys were found to fire identically when the animal grasped a peanut and when it watched another monkey do the same. The monkey's brain was acting as if it were picking up the peanut even though it was merely observing another monkey doing so. The finding sparked the interest of scientists all over the world, spawning a considerable amount of research on whether human beings also possess these so-called mirror neurons. We now know that we do. We also know that the human variety is much more sophisticated, able to mirror not only the movements of others but their emotions and feelings as well. When others move, we move (in our minds, that is). When others are happy or sad, we are happy or sad (again, not literally, but in our minds, which are simulating their emotions).

Clearly the brain's mirroring system must contribute to the profoundly social nature of human beings. Philosophers who spoke of existence as a being-in-the-world now appear to have been quite prescient. Our minds *are* constantly connecting us to other people—to their actions, emotions, and thoughts—connecting and at the same time synchronizing us in even more visceral ways than Merleau-Ponty and others might have imagined. But why? Though the science is still in its early stages, researchers believe that neuronal mirroring plays a critical role in how human beings live and work together so much more successfully than our evolutionary predecessors did. It may in fact be responsible for some of our greatest collective achievements: language, social institutions, culture. Imitating the facial movements of an adult who is speaking, for example, may help a child learn to speak. Similar processes may enable us to interpret the intentions behind other people's actions ("reading" their minds) and to empathize with other people's feelings (prompting the scientist V. S. Ramachandran to refer to our Dalai Lama neurons).

Many scientists also believe that the brain's mirroring system can reflect in two directions, illuminating not just the outside world (of others) but the inside world (of self). Again the philosophers' speculations seem to have been right on target, for existence, phenomenological and now physiological, *is* turning out to be a dialogue with the world—we listen and respond to it, and it listens and responds to us. By observing and imitating others, we learn not only about them but also about ourselves: how we see and think of ourselves and the meanings we ultimately give to our most subjective experiences, like pain. Isn't that why patients, who despite their feelings of inwardness and isolation, continue to seek out doppelgangers? Certainly they wish to validate their experiences and find sympathy. But aren't they also motivated to see and learn about themselves?

Frigyes Karinthy was a well-known Hungarian writer of the early twentieth century who developed a brain tumor. The tumor was diagnosed not by one of the many specialists he consulted but rather, quite remarkably, by himself, a layman who never went to medical school. He did so with the help of a metaphorical mirror.

The first clue came when he began hearing trains in his head. Next came the giddy sensations of pictures and tables moving slightly one way and then back again. Then there were headaches and fainting fits. One doctor attributed the symptoms to an ear infection, another to nicotine poisoning, and a third to humiliations suffered in early childhood. In each case, none of the prescribed interventions helped, and for a while Karinthy was determined to live with the trains and hallucinations, denying their importance as his doctors did. But when they persisted and new symptoms developed, he could deny them no longer. They were interfering with every aspect of his life. Regardless of what the doctors thought, something was wrong—very wrong.

Proof of his conviction came serendipitously. Karinthy was visiting the clinic where his wife, a doctor, worked. Accompanying her on rounds, Karinthy stopped at the bed of a young man, transfixed by the expression on his face. It looked familiar, he thought. *The man has a brain tumor*, his wife grimly informed him, *and is terminal*. Ah, Karinthy remembered, he *had* seen that face before, in a friend who had died many years before of the same condition. But Karinthy wasn't entirely satisfied. He continued to be haunted by the sight. It reminded him of someone else too, he was sure.

Later on, it hit him with the full force of the roaring trains in his head:

> I had suddenly stopped dead in the gateway, like the ox I had seen unwilling to enter the slaughter-house. At that moment, it had flashed into my mind. I remembered. The pale, vacant face of the dying man reminded me of my own expression as I had seen it lately in my mirror while shaving. I took two steps, then stopped again. With a foolish grimace, like a man who pretends to belittle some achievement he is boasting about, I said to my wife:
>
> "Aranka, I've got a tumor on the brain."

Aranka dismissed her husband's epiphany as crazy. But she was soon proven wrong. Fortunately, things would turn out well for Karinthy. He was successfully operated on by the famous Swedish neurosurgeon Olivecrona. Afterward he returned to his writing career and published his best work, a memoir of his fascinating encounter with illness, *A Journey Round My Skull*.

If the scientists are right about mirror neurons, then perhaps we really are hardwired to see ourselves in other patients, literally with our eyes and more figuratively with our mind's eye. We are hardwired, too, to see ourselves in the fictional characters of the books we read and the movies we watch, and to see ourselves even in things that are not like us—a solitary seal or a struggling tree. But having a genetic predisposition doesn't mean that the seeing is necessarily a passive, automatic activity (the way the heart beats, lungs expand, and most mirror neurons seem to work). As Nelson Goodman observes in *Ways of Worldmaking*, if the seeing leads to a change in the way we understand the world, then it requires work on our part. Karinthy, for example, instantly saw the patient's expression but didn't recognize himself in it until he had reproduced the expression in his brain via mirror neurons and then compared it with memories of his friend. Insight came when Karinthy identified and imposed a pattern on the different strands of incoming data.

> If worlds are made as much as found, so also knowing is as much remaking as reporting. All the processes of worldmaking I have discussed enter into knowing. Perceiving motion, we have seen, often consists in producing it. Discovering laws involves drafting them. Recognizing patterns is very much a matter of inventing and imposing them. *Comprehension and creation go on together.* [my italics]

Mimesis may be a prerequisite or stepping-stone to knowledge. We observe, reproduce, impose patterns, and thereby understand. We do this with objects that happen to cross our field of vision, like the seal encountered by Mark Doty or the patient encountered by Frigyes Karinthy. But we could also do this on a more sophisticated level through metaphor. If a potential copy or doppelganger doesn't exist, we can invent one, as Daudet does in his dream of the damaged boat or as artists do in their poems and paintings. After finishing his masterwork, Gustave Flaubert is famously reported to have said of his creation, *"Emma Bovary, c'est moi."* The reproduction leads to recognition, as it does more self-consciously for painters in their self-portraits, and in the case of Frida Kahlo, double self-portraits. In *The Two Fridas*, the mirror of Kahlo's imagination produces two very different images of herself: one European, formal, and mortally wounded

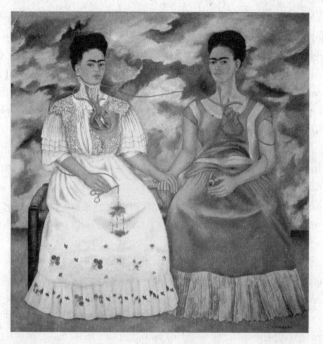

The Two Fridas by Frida Kahlo. © *2009 Banco de Mexico Diego Rivera Frida Kahlo Museums Trust, Mexico, D.F. / Artists Rights Society (ARS).*

by her husband's infidelity; the other Mexican, more relaxed, not wounded and still loved. The alter egos, however, support each other, physically through the commingling of blood and emotionally by the holding of hands, and together make up a unified Frida.

In examples such as these, Goodman's dictum is most transparently realized: comprehension and creation go on together.

THE MADE WORLD AS MIRROR

Perhaps projection is simply a higher-order version of neuronal mirroring. We learn about others and ourselves through the unconscious activity of certain neurons and also through the more conscious activity of the imaginative centers in the brain. We *intentionally* recreate ourselves in the world around us by projecting our feelings and thoughts onto external objects. The world in a sense becomes our mirror. For Elaine Scarry this trajectory is central to all creative acts. Whenever we make something—a chair, a house, a poem—we thrust our entire selves into the making, not just physically but through the desires and other feelings that motivate us to create in the first place. Moreover, this projection of human sentience leaves a permanent residue in the finished product. Artifacts, by their very nature, are saturated with what it means and feels like to be human.

This human residue is most apparent when it appears on the surface of made objects, many of which quite literally mirror us. A shirt bears the shape of our upper body. Eyeglasses remind us of the eyes. On a more abstract level, the made world mirrors certain human capacities and needs. The photocopier reflects our capacity to remember, clothes reflect our capacity to keep our bodies warm, chairs reflect our desire to relieve the burden of weight. More abstract still, the artifact at times radiates the most basic property of lived existence, our aliveness. A cane, we might remember, can become so much a part of us that it seems to "feel" the pavement as our feet do and perhaps even "feel pain" as we might when something smashes into it (and us).

As Scarry eloquently suggests, the dividends of this personal investment are enormous. We project ourselves into the things we make for good reason: now those things can work for us. Artifacts, for example, can help us realize all the important goals we attributed to literary projection. They can validate our most personal experiences by shifting their existence from the private to the public world. The McGill Pain Questionnaire not only helps patients describe their pain but also substantiates the reality of their pain. So do the striking images of suffering created by Munch and Kahlo. At the same time, creation works to fill the world with sympathetic and responsive objects. In addition to the natural world of rivers and mountains and skies, which are indifferent to human sentience, there are now numerous made objects that are inherently "mindful" of us—the lighthouse that guides the terrified survivors of ship-wrecks back to safety, the songs and paintings that mime and "under-stand" our pain.

What's more, this mindfulness often exceeds the mindfulness that comes from other human beings, our doctors and even our friends. The artifact doesn't depend on the presence and goodwill of others, who may or may not believe our pain. Nor is it temporally bounded, like a human response. The chair that supports a pregnant woman contains within its very structure a sustained expression of the willingness to take on her weight, as well as that of anyone else who reclines in its comfort. It no longer matters whether the woman has a compassionate husband, an indifferent one, or a malicious one. "The general distribution of material objects to a population," writes Scarry, "means that a certain minimum level of objectified human compassion is built into the revised structure of the external world, and does not depend on the day-by-day generosity of other inhabitants which itself cannot be legislated."

Finally, we invest ourselves in acts of creation in order to enhance ourselves. Eyeglasses don't just mime the eyes, they improve them. Similarly, the photocopier and computer improve our capacity to remember, and the telephone accommodates our ability and desire to speak to people across great distances. In addition, by enhancing our eyesight, eyeglasses relieve us of the need to worry about our defec-tive vision (and the unpleasant sensations it causes) so that we can attend to other things. In this way, the material world can be said to disembody us, to free us from what would otherwise be an over-whelming and ongoing preoccupation with our bodies. To use Scar-ry's example:

The simple triad of floor, chair, and bed (or simpler still, floor, stool, and mat) makes spatially and therefore steadily visible the collection of postures and positions the body moves in and out of, objectifies the three locations that most frequently hold the body's weight, objectifies its need continually to shift within itself the locus of its weight, objectifies, finally, its need to become wholly forgetful of its weight, to move weightlessly into a larger mindfulness.

No wonder, then, that artifacts assume such significance for the sufferers in the stories of London, Tolstoy, and Crane. Immersed in the isolating epoché of pain, these men and women embrace the slightest shred of the material world that appears before them. Crane's survivors enlarge, color, and fill in every gap until the point they see at the horizon turns into a lighthouse. Tolstoy's character squints and strains until the haziness of the white waste materializes into another carriage or a nearby village. The artifact is metonymic of the world that is no longer with them; it carries in its wake the rest of human civilization. Moreover, the artifact is imbued with the collective sentience built into that civilization. The lighthouse, the carriage, the village—all possess a voice that enables them to speak to the sufferer: *We have been created for your use*, they say; *we recognize the danger you now face and we are concerned*. In a way, there is no need to imagine these objects entering into conversation with human beings, as we did with the hyena or willow trees; they do so almost literally.

For these reasons, the artifact is a natural fit for projection metaphors used to represent pain. Consider the house occupied by former slaves in Morrison's *Beloved*: 124, as it is called, is almost never regarded as a thing but as a person—a person with a history of "unspeakable" suffering that it shares with the people who live within its walls. There should be no surprise, then, that the house begins to weep and sigh and tremble; or that it remains isolated from the rest of the town because no one ever comes to visit; or that Paul D, when he enters for the first time, describes it as sad and soaked with grief. The house *is* as lonely and sad as Sethe, Denver, and Baby Suggs before she died. And haunted too, as Morrison continues to push the metaphor forward, by the painful memories of Sethe's other daughter, whom she killed to protect from becoming a slave. Initially the presence of those memories is felt only indirectly, in undulating red lights and grinding floorboards. Later on, however, they materialize into a full-fledged, insatiable ghost that feeds on and destroys the living (like guilt and grief). In these ways, Morrison works to transform 124 into a visible and articulate record of the suffering, past and present, of its inhabitants.

In "Master and Man" we find another artifact that is used to create a compelling projection metaphor: clothing. At the beginning of the story, Tolstoy points out that what a person wears can tell us much about his wealth and social status. Master Vasili appears quite comfortable in his "cloth-covered sheepskin coat tightly girdled low at his waist," his felt boots with leather soles, and his thick padded gloves. Servant Nikita, in contrast, is dressed in a short coat "torn under the arms and at the back, greasy and out of shape, and frayed to a fringe round the skirt." Vasili can only laugh when he sees the pitiful outfit.

During their fateful journey, however, Vasili's attitude radically changes. As he begins to suffer, he realizes that his superior outerwear cannot shield him from the cold, which penetrates right through and causes him pain:

> His body, especially between his legs where it touched the pad of the harness and was not covered by his overcoats, was getting painfully cold. . . . His legs and arms trembled and his breathing came fast. . . . It was real snow that lashed his face and covered him and chilled his right hand from which he had lost the glove.

Vasili's clothing—its limitations—makes him aware of the body's fragility. He may not be as different from Nikita as he had previously imagined. In the end their bodies hurt in the same way.

His thoughts are further clarified when he encounters several articles of frozen clothing on a line behind one of the houses in the village. Like the sequence of the wormwood trees, the reappearance of the clothesline on four distinct occasions serves to focus Vasili's attention on the body in pain. He spots the line during their first pass through the village:

> At the end house of the village some frozen clothes hanging on a line—shirts, one red and one white, trousers, leg-bands, and a petticoat—fluttered wildly in the wind. The white shirt in particular struggled desperately, waving its sleeves about.

With a little imagination, Vasili can join the pieces of clothing together to "recreate" the human form—pants as legs, sleeves as arms. He might also recognize in the artifacts a specific capacity or need of the body—the need, as he appreciates now more than ever, to maintain a stable internal temperature. And last, the clothing may remind him of the essence of the body's interior, its aliveness. The shirt, becoming animated, is pictured as struggling and waving its sleeves about.

Passing the village a second time, Vasili sees the line again. One of the shirts has become detached and is clinging for dear life:

> Past the yard where the clothes hung out . . . the white shirt had broken loose and was now attached only by one frozen sleeve.

On the third pass, the frozen clothing continues to flutter "desperately in the wind." And on the fourth and final pass, the clothesline is empty.

Like the wormwood trees, the clothes are credited with the capacity to feel pain. But while human pain resides in an inaccessible interior, the artifact's pain resides on its surface. Vasili can see, touch, and hear it. When at last he discovers himself in the artifact—the clothes struggle desperately to stave off the cold, just as he does; they freeze the same way he does; and when pieced together, they look just like him—Vasili finally understands what it means to suffer and how indifferent he has been to the suffering around him. Acknowledging pain's aversiveness, he can no longer look on passively but must act. In a grand Tolstoyan stroke of redemption, Vasili uses his body as a piece of clothing, covering Nikita's body so that he can preserve his servant's threatened core temperature while disregarding his own.

Vasili Andreevich stood silent and motionless for half a minute. Then suddenly, with the same resolution with which he used to strike hands when making a good purchase, he took a step back and turning up his sleeves began raking the snow off Nikita and out of the sledge. Having done this he hurriedly undid his girdle, opened out his fur coat, and having pushed Nikita down, lay down on top of him, covering him not only with his fur coat but with the whole of his body, which glowed with warmth.

Another fascinating example of an artifact that mirrors human suffering occurs in Crane's "The Open Boat," as the survivors become progressively inseparable (and indistinguishable) from their boat. At the outset of the story, the ocean is identified as an agent as it moves against the men threateningly and voices its hostility. But an actual collision never takes place. Protectively mediating between ocean and sufferer, the boat becomes an additional outer layer or extension of the human body. It bears the brunt of the agent's force and at the same time enables the survivors to observe that force and its potential to damage and inflict pain on material objects in its path.

Initially we learn that the captain is "rooted deep" within the dinghy's timbers. The rest of the crew experience a similarly visceral involvement as they must synchronize their movements with the boat's. When a gull sets down on the bow, the captain doesn't dare wave it away, "because anything resembling an emphatic gesture would have capsized the freighted boat." Despite the pain that arises from their immobility, the men must relinquish the claims of their own bodies for the body of the artifact.

Gradually the dinghy begins to acquire the physical form and behavior of its occupants. The captain removes his overcoat and uses it as a sail. The boat, no longer a collection of inanimate timbers, becomes alive: "The craft pranced and reared, and plunged like an animal." And since it looks and acts like a human being, then perhaps the boat also feels pain and deserves our sympathy:

> But the waves continued their old impetuous swooping at the dinghy, and the little craft, no longer under way, struggled woundily over them.

> The little boat . . . splashed viciously by the crests. . . . She seemed just a wee thing wallowing, miraculously, top-up, at the mercy of the five oceans.

The metaphoric dialogue between human being and artifact enables the sufferer (or the author on his behalf) to represent how he feels effectively. Unlike the invisible and indeterminate quality of pain, the wounded dinghy can be seen by and talked about with other people.

Even more remarkable about the representation is its elimination of the actual sufferer. Who, in fact, is *struggling woundily*? Who is wallowing at the mercy of the ocean? Completely intertwined with the survivors, the dinghy becomes the sole entity that experiences pain and demands our pity. Meanwhile the survivors are gradually removed from the event and transformed into observers. By redirecting the agent against the boat, they not only are able to visualize their suffering but actually begin to diminish it. Creation, whether in the form of medicine or metaphor, disembodies us, divests us of a sentience that at times can be overwhelming.

Appropriately, the projection metaphor effectively captures—better yet, mirrors—our desire to end the pain we feel. It also captures our equally strong desire to end the pain we observe in another. As Scarry recognizes, it is practically impossible to witness someone else's pain without wishing it gone:

> If one imagines one human being seeing another human being in pain, one human being perceiving in another discomfort and in

the same moment wishing the other to be relieved of the discomfort, something in that fraction of a second is occurring inside the first person's brain involving the complex action of many neurons that is, importantly, not just a perception of an actuality (the second person's pain) but an alteration of that actuality (for embedded in the perception is the sorrow that it is so, the wish that it were otherwise). Though this interior event must be expressed as a conjunctive duality, "seeing the pain and wishing it gone," it is a single percipient event in which the reality of pain and the unreality of imagining are already conflated. Neither can occur without the other: if the person does not perceive the distress, neither will he wish it gone; conversely, if he does not wish it gone, he cannot have perceived the pain itself.

Remaking pain by picturing an agent harming a surrogate body elegantly captures this conjunctive duality. It enables both sufferer and observer to perceive the event while desiring to radically alter it. In the same way, Alphonse Daudet disperses some of his pain onto his fellow sufferers at Lamalou and some onto the injured boat in his dreams. And in the same way, Christian Wiman shares his pain with the apple sapling in his backyard. Like characters in fiction, real patients are drawn to projection metaphors for the same reason they are drawn to medicine: to alleviate their pain.

The human mind operates like a mirror. It can do so directly (Karinthy recognizing himself in another patient) or indirectly (Crane's survivors recognizing themselves in a boat). While the latter instances may require more creative and imaginative effort on the part of the sufferer, they offer significant advantages over the former. First, the more patently metaphorical projections don't depend on the presence of other people; we may not always be lucky enough to encounter a real-life doppelganger. And second, they don't depend on the existence of additional suffering, whether that of other people or of ourselves. We may not need another brain-tumor patient to see ourselves as a brain-tumor patient. We may not need to slash our arms like the woman from the pain clinic in order to validate and mirror the pain we feel inside. Instead, we can create surrogate and imagined sufferers that suffer with and perhaps for us, like Morrison's house, Tolstoy's clothes, and Crane's boat.

While in this last section we have been explicitly focusing on the dialogue between artifact and sufferer, the fact is that all the objects that serve as vehicles in projection metaphors—hyena, seal, rooster, willow trees, apple sapling—are themselves artifacts. On the one hand, they are parts of the larger artifact of the literary text, a text made up of words on paper and created by a writer to convey the suffering of real or imagined people to an audience of readers. On a second level, within the text, those people are themselves engaged in understanding and conveying their pain. They succeed by interacting with objects in their environment—that is, the characters "artifactualize" or remake these objects by imagining them to possess human sentience.

By examining stories about pain (artifact as product) and the language employed by the characters in these stories (artifact in the process of production), we have the opportunity to see things from an omniscient point of view—to see pain from the perspective of both the sufferer and the observer; to see it, that is, from the inside and the outside simultaneously. The sufferers, severed from the world, urgently wish to understand what is occurring within them, to free themselves from the body's concerns and reintegrate themselves into a world more responsive to their needs. Observers, however, must be made to perceive the pain of others so that there is no possible way of dismissing it; they must be made to recognize both the sufferers' attempt to understand the body in pain and their need to transcend it. Projection metaphors, like the language of agency, are linguistic strategies or verbal artifacts created to meet the demands of both parties.

The X-Ray

The ocean drained like a bathtub and showed its
insides, its seaweed and mussels and clams and
creatures, exposing all the subtle movement and life
of its body beneath the skin, inviting exploration of
its most private places.

—NELLIE HERMANN, *The Cure for Grief*

Hans Castorp lives in the bustling port city of Hamburg. He
is young, healthy, enthusiastic, and about to embark on a successful career in the family business, shipping. There's nowhere to
go but up.

That is until a visit to Davos, Switzerland, to see his sick cousin
turns into a seven-year stay that radically alters the course of Hans's
trajectory. At the Magic Mountain he encounters what Susan Sontag once called the "night-side" of life—illness and the far-reaching
consequences it has on a person.

To get there, Hans must physically journey up into the mountains. But the night side of life is also figuratively remote from the
day side. When healthy, one focuses almost exclusively on the world
of other people and things—on appearances, money, advancement,
status. The sick, however, turn inward, unable to focus on anything
but themselves and their bodies. At first Hans witnesses the rumblings of the sick body from a distance, in the symptoms of the
patients he meets. There is, for example, the cough of the gentleman rider:

It was coughing . . . like to no other Hans Castorp had ever heard, and compared with which any other had been a magnificent and healthy manifestation of life. . . . It isn't a human cough at all.

What Hans finds strange is not so much the cough but what it stands for, the cough as a sign of disease lurking beneath the surface. When he hears it, he feels as if he could peer right into the man's body and see the "feeble, dreadful welling up of the juices of organic dissolution . . . all slime and mucous."

Soon Hans develops his own symptoms. He has fevers and palpitations. Later he begins to cough like the gentleman rider and other tuberculosis patients at the sanatorium. At first he isn't upset. Indeed, at times when he feels most sick, he is moved by an "extravagant thrill of joy" and "a feeling of reckless sweetness." No doubt the signs emanating from the body's depths are novel and mysterious to Hans. They promise him adventure, maybe even passion.

But the desire to journey into the uncharted landscape of the body is hard to satisfy. For most of us, the body's interior is a black box filled with vague contents. What is causing the fever and the cough? What is happening inside that triggers the strange sensations? How will it turn out? These are questions every patient asks, and the desire to know only grows as the disease progresses, ultimately triggering another common feeling among patients: frustration.

A turning point comes when Hans visits the radiology department and is shown the source of his symptoms. There in the dimly lit room, the black box of his interior is illuminated by the X-ray. No longer remote and hazy, the body is now grasped in a concrete and palpable way. He sees the bones in his hand, the rib cage encircling the chest. He sees the tubercular strands and nodules in his lungs. Afterward, the radiologist lets him watch his cousin's heart in action, as it expands and contracts like a "swimming jellyfish."

And Hans Castorp saw, precisely what he must have expected, but what it is hardly permitted man to see, and what he had never thought it would be vouchsafed for him to see: he looked into his own grave. The process of decay was forestalled by the powers of the light ray, the flesh in which he walked disintegrated, annihilated, dissolved in vacant mist . . . he gazed at the familiar part of his own body, and for the first time in his life he understood that he would die.

Although this new knowledge of the body's interior is unsettling, it nonetheless helps Hans throughout his stay at Davos. It enables him to make sense of what is happening to him in a way that he couldn't before. Hans keeps the X-ray copy in his breast pocket as a memento mori. Whenever he feels his heart pounding, he thinks of the swimming jellyfish. Whenever he coughs, he recalls the strands and nodules in his lungs. Now he not only hears the inarticulate voice of the body but also begins to grasp its internal mechanisms that work to keep him alive.

The personal gain in knowledge for Hans Castorp, Thomas Mann's character in *The Magic Mountain*, recalls the more universal gains for Bichat and his colleagues in France at the turn of the nineteenth century. As Foucault reminds us, they too were frustrated by their inability to understand the body in disease, and for the same reason: they couldn't see it. Only the French physicians responded in a much more radical way, by blasting open the black box and peeling back the surface. Once this was done, they could begin to study the body in a systematic way. Thus the field of pathological anatomy was born.

The work of the French physicians underscores the importance of perception, especially vision, to the acquisition of knowledge. Once we can *see* something, we can talk about and try to understand it. As Foucault says, the making visible leads to a making *dicible* (sayable) and *discible* (learnable). This is why we speak interchangeably of knowledge and illumination or insight. It also brings us to the third strategy used to represent the felt experience of pain. Instead of literally opening up corpses or looking into the body with one of modern medicine's many imaging techniques (X-ray, CAT scan, MRI), we can imagine and picture its interior landscape with words and metaphor.

IMAGING THE BODY

Before turning to examples of this kind of metaphorical introspection, we should once again remind ourselves of the project's intrinsic difficulties. We can't ordinarily see (or taste, hear, smell, touch) most of the body's interior; perception, as we said, is primarily perception of the external world. And the sensations that do come to us from the interior provide minimal information. As incontestably real and immediate as twinges, itches, aches, and pains are, they lack the clarity and determinacy of perceptual experience (seeing a bird, for example, and listening to its call). This haziness, we have noted, can be attributed to the absence of recognizable sensory organs inside the body; the lack of control over how sensations are registered (we can't muffle or shade them as we can external sounds and sights); and our inability to confer with others about their nature (we can't ask someone about a twinge in our leg as we might about a bird passing overhead).

But disregarding how little we know of the body's interior, the vast majority of what happens there is *not experienced at all*. We neither feel nor are aware of most events that take place in our organs and tissues, within the individual cells of those organs, and, more remote still, at the molecular level within those cells. When Hans Castorp travels to the Magic Mountain, he probably develops altitude sickness and what physicians call its nonspecific symptoms (lightheadedness, dizziness, and nausea). But Hans would be hard-pressed to describe the sensations and explain their significance. Nevertheless, while he remains relatively oblivious, his body registers and responds to the altitude change in exquisitely specific and precise ways. Special sensors in the carotid artery detect the higher altitude because of lower oxygen levels in the blood. Hypoxia in turn generates higher respiratory rates, increased production of hemoglobin (the protein in red blood cells that binds oxygen), and a decreased affinity between hemoglobin and oxygen (so that more oxygen can be released to hypoxic tissues). These responses, all of which take place involuntarily and unconsciously, enable the body to maintain its interior equilibrium, or homeostasis.

Our relative detachment from the body should not be considered a flaw or accident in its design but rather its intent. Imagine if we had to concentrate on breathing every second of the day, or if we had to think about ratcheting up our heartrate during exercise or coaxing hemoglobin molecules to let go of oxygen at higher altitudes. Imagine if every slight alteration inside the body were felt. It would drive us insane, or at the very least distract us. Thankfully, the body runs for the most part automatically and silently. This characteristic not only preserves our sanity but also allows us to focus on our main priority—the world beyond the body. Survival depends on being able to recognize the threats and opportunities in the external world, which is ultimately why the normal perspective of existence must be outward-facing, a being-in-the-world.

All this changes, however, when we are ill and in pain. Here our priorities radically shift. The inside world (where the main threat now lies) becomes more important than the outside one, and more vocal. As those previously quiet inner processes are disrupted and begin to fail, they become noisy and demand our attention. When the tubercle bacillus invades Hans's lungs, causing him to cough and wheeze, he can't help but focus on the act of breathing. Nor can he continue, as he did in Hamburg when healthy, to pursue his great ambitions in the world. No longer relieved of bodily sentience, he remains in the most unproductive of states.

As we might expect, this unfamiliar shift in perspective presents a problem, for the body remains as opaque in illness as it is in health. Although it "wells up" and demands to be heard, what do we hear? What can we see? Not very much. Initially this may not be distressing. For Hans, remember, there is a new and adventurous side to joining the tuberculosis club at the Magic Mountain. But the novelty quickly fades as the symptoms and threat level mount: when you can't move and are confined to a bed; when breathing becomes increasingly labored or the pain just won't go away; or when, even in the absence of physical symptoms, a dire diagnosis is made—when lung or breast cancer is detected on a routine X-ray. Then you can no longer look the other way or spin the facts in a positive light. Now it is much too serious. We can't help but want to see what's happening, to find out why, and to plan a strategy for dealing with the threat. We must have answers.

Hans is fortunate in this regard. He has doctors who understand his needs, guide him through the unfamiliar terrain of tuberculosis, and illuminate its salient features. The images of and explanations about his diseased lungs are a great comfort to him during his illness. But Hans's case is not the norm. Most patients don't receive this degree of attention from their doctors. And the information they may find in the library or on the Internet isn't always satisfying. It may be difficult to interpret and is often overly abstract and impersonal. We all need something simpler and more clear-cut, even doctors who become patients, like myself. In these instances we will do what the characters in the stories do—we will illuminate what is happening inside the body on our own, using pictures and metaphors. Although our experience of the body is "so vague and muddy," writes the physician and polymath Jonathan Miller,

> our mind does everything it can to intensify the images with which it is supplied. . . . In the absence of any immediate knowledge of our insides, most of us have improvised an imaginary picture in the hope of explaining the occasional feelings which escape into consciousness. Our mind, it seems, prefers a picture of some sort to having to live through the chaos of sensations that would otherwise seem absurd.

Such pictures are invaluable in the crisis settings of illness and pain. They make our experiences, all-consuming yet excessively vague, more palpably real for us. They also make them more meaningful.

I relied on pictures during my hospitalization almost as much as I relied on my family and narcotics. Just before my transplant, after a week of intensive chemotherapy and radiation, the lining of my gastrointestinal tract begin to slough, leaving me with a string of ulcers from the mouth to the anus. The pain was unbearable. Yet as much as I wanted to close my eyes and never wake up, I couldn't ignore what was happening. I had to see it. So in my mind's eye I pictured a forest fire sweeping down the long and convoluted underground piping network of my digestive tract—a combination of agent and anatomic metaphors. The image was a more disseminated version of what frequently appears in pharmaceutical advertisements for peptic ulcer disease. Like those ads, the picture not only helped me think and talk about my pain but, equally important, suggested ways of responding to it. I needed medicine that could put out stomach fires or someone who could literally hose me down—which is precisely what the all-knowing gods at Memorial Sloan-Kettering Cancer Center beneficently provided for their transplant patients. Every day a nurse I came to call the Rinser would squirt water down my throat for twenty minutes at a time. And when the Rinser was elsewhere or the morphine inadequate, I would make do with my pictures—now a cool and endless stream of water flowing over and dampening the smoldering fires, allowing my mucosal cells to heal. A mind game, perhaps, but one that helped me considerably, as it does many patients.

Frida Kahlo may be the best example of a patient who created pictures to relieve her suffering. The great Mexican artist lived most of her life in pain. As a child she developed polio and was confined to her room for almost a year. At fifteen she was involved in a horrendous bus accident in which she fractured her spinal column (in three places), her collarbone, several ribs, and several bones in her right foot. The accident led to ongoing pain, ongoing confinement—

for herself (in hospitals) and for parts of her body (in casts and corsets)—and more than thirty-two surgical operations to repair the damage. Beyond this, she had problems with her husband, the artist Diego Rivera, and went through several agonizing and unsuccessful attempts to have a child.

Kahlo also spent most of her life trying to make sense of her pain, trying to answer the "what" and the "why" questions that plague so many patients. Because her gift was more visual than verbal, she tried to answer these questions in her paintings, images that offer us a unique opportunity to witness some of the most articulate representations of suffering ever created.

Kahlo used many of the strategies discussed in this book. She used images of weapons (knives, swords, and arrows) and wounds that are characteristic of the agency metaphor in paintings titled *Memory, Remembrance of an Open Wound,* and *A Few Small Nips.* She also projected her feelings onto other objects, picturing her fractured body in a fractured landscape (*Tree of Hope*) and imagining herself as a wounded deer (*The Little Deer*). The self-duplications in many of her paintings (*The Two Fridas, The Dream, Tree of Hope*) are also examples of projection metaphors. In these variations on traditional self-portraiture, Kahlo is able not only to view herself from the outside, creating what Alphonse Daudet called a doppelganger of pain, but also to express contrasting feelings simultaneously. She paints what she sees in the mirror and what she desires to see in the mirror. In the process, she gains instant companionship and a better understanding of her pain, which she can then share with others.

Perhaps the most remarkable images of all are those in which Kahlo's desire to know prompts her to probe even deeper, to search for the origins of her pain. Like Foucault's French physicians, Kahlo isn't satisfied with observing merely the outer surface of the body; she wants to see and make sense of what is happening inside; she wants to illuminate the source of her pain. So she too begins to pry open the black box.

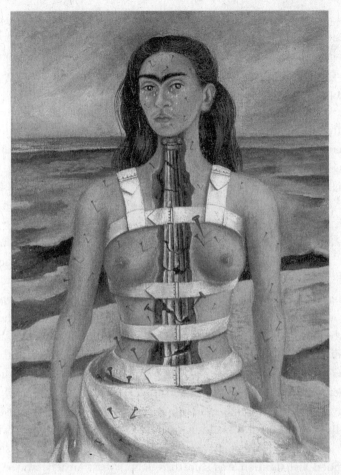

Broken Column by Frida Kahlo. © 2009 *Banco de Mexico Diego Rivera Frida Kahlo Museums Trust, Mexico, D.F. / Artists Rights Society (ARS).*

In *The Broken Column*, Kahlo's naked body is dissected down the middle, exposing an Ionic column that is cracked at numerous points. A stiff, sturdy corset holds the crumbling column-spine together. The corset also helps the spine perform one of its primary functions, to keep the body erect. The nails piercing the body convey the depth of the pain experienced by the artist.

Like many of Kahlo's works, this is a disturbing image, yet it has a positive and therapeutic role. Kahlo's artistic gift enables her to replace the darkness and mystery of the body with a picture, one that gives her experience a clarity and coherence it would otherwise not possess while, at the same time, shifting it from an inner, private one to an outer, public one. Anyone who looks at Kahlo's art has a better understanding of her suffering. "My painting," she told a friend just before she died, "carries within it the message of pain." The picture also contains an effective response to her suffering, for what she envisioned in her imagination—easing pain by buttressing her damaged spine—has now materialized before her. She literally can *see* her pain being diminished.

Not everyone is as talented as Frida Kahlo, capable of creating such expressive pictures. But they can be nudged. Several decades ago, oncologists and other health-care providers introduced guided imagery and visualization techniques into the therapeutic arsenal. Drawing on Eastern religious and philosophical traditions, these techniques sought to harness the powers of the mind to help the body fight disease. Patients were first taught how to relax and then encouraged to imagine what was happening inside their bodies. They would draw themselves and their cancers. Next they would draw how their treatment and immune cells fought their cancers, as in the picture below, made by a thirty-three-year-old woman with breast cancer. The benefits of such therapy were often impressive. Guided visualization was said to reduce stress, anxiety, and even pain to a certain degree.

Nowadays almost every major cancer center in the United States has an art therapy program. Similar programs have sprouted up for patients with just about every other medical condition. In contrast to earlier versions, the current emphasis of art therapy is on expression as an end in itself rather than as a means toward more favorable outcomes. Naturally, therapists hope that patients will fare better if they can communicate more effectively and feel less isolated. But they don't want to place an additional burden on patients by making them feel as if they are responsible for the outcomes of

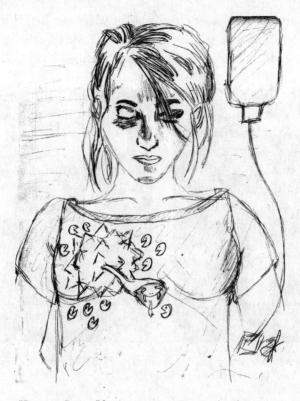

"Serpent Cancer" by Anonymous. *Reprinted with permission from the artist.*

their illnesses—if their cancer-fighting immune cells, for example, appear too weak or if their drawings reveal a negative attitude.

One of the most exciting recent projects in the field is the artist Deborah Padfield's work with patients at a pain clinic in England. A chronic pain patient herself, Padfield understands all too well the frustration of her fellow sufferers—that because their pain has gone unheard for so long, it begins to seem more and more unreal, both to themselves and to others. Padfield created photographic images and collages in collaboration with patients that were able to illuminate their increasingly distant and lonely worlds, to make, in Styron's words, "the darkness visible." Not surprisingly, weapons figure prominently in these images. One patient with pain for forty-two years described the sensation as "red hot swords on fire" that constantly rip down her leg. "If I could get my hand in, I could lift it out," she tells Padfield. "I could rip it out, it is so specific."

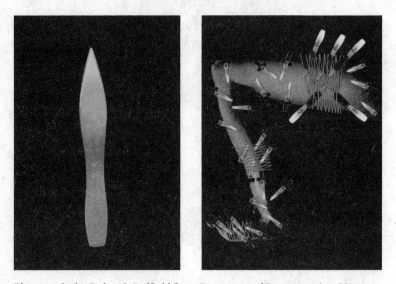

Photographs by Deborah Padfield from *Perceptions of Pain. Reproduced by permission of Dewi Lewis Publishing, Stockport, UK, 2003.*

There are also many instances when patients looked further inward, imagining what was taking place beneath their skin. One man described his pain as an intense coldness growing in his limbs, as if his veins were beginning to freeze and his whole body might turn into a block of ice. A sufferer with polio had trouble breathing. Like London's hurricane victims, he imagined a dense substance clogging up his airways. He decided there was a cement mixer in his chest, which produced a substance that would harden and prevent his lungs from expanding and contracting (and him from inhaling and exhaling).

The photographic collages were uniformly revealing and liberating for Padfield's fellow sufferers. "When I first saw the images that Deborah and I produced together, I felt a shiver of recognition filled

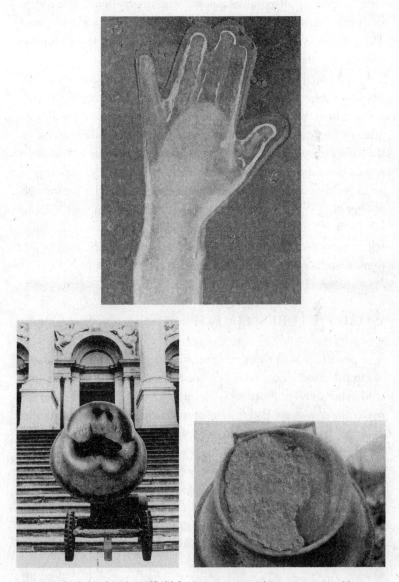

Photographs by Deborah Padfield from *Perceptions of Pain*. *Reproduced by permission of Dewi Lewis Publishing, Stockport, UK, 2003.*

with feelings of anger and sadness," said one patient. "But for the first time I was able to point at something and say 'that's my pain.'" The collages were also helpful to the doctors at the clinic, for now they could better understand their patients' pain.

Like Frida Kahlo, patients must be able to express how they feel. They must be able to give their experiences form and meaning in whatever medium they are comfortable with. If they can't find words, then perhaps they can make pictures. Either route allows them to escape the isolating epoché of pain. Expression inevitably leads to knowledge and community, and it may also work like medicine to lessen our pain, as my pictures did for me in the hospital and Frida's did for her throughout her life. "When I wake up at night in pain now," another of Deborah Padfield's patient-collaborators said with a confidence she hadn't felt in years, "instead of feeling controlled and overwhelmed by it, I think about how I might represent it visually."

WORD PICTURES: SIMPLE

If, as Jonathan Miller suggests, we prefer pictures to the muddiness of internal experience, we needn't restrict ourselves to images generated in our mind or those we draw on paper and canvas. We can also make pictures of the body's interior with words, what we have called anatomic metaphors. In a sense, these metaphors reverse the direction of projection metaphors; instead of moving our inside world outside (projecting our feelings onto external objects), we now move the outside world inside (bringing external objects into the body). This is what James Joyce did when his young alter ego fell ill at boarding school. He imagined a faucet inside Stephen Dedalus's body that alternately ran hot and cold water and a train that passed through the tunnel of his ear, roaring and stopping.

Like Joyce, Tolstoy used anatomic metaphors to represent the pain of his characters. In "How Much Land Does a Man Need?," we encounter a Russian merchant who may be even greedier than Vasili

from "Master and Man." Pakhom is promised all the land he can tra-
verse by foot in a single day as long as he is able to return to the
starting point before sunset. Predictably, his desire for great wealth
causes him to misjudge the distance he has traveled and the time it
will take to get back. He also ignores the physical demands of the
journey on his body. At the end of the day, when exhaustion and pain
set in, however, Pakhom's perspective abruptly shifts. Where formerly
he focused on what lay before him—land, money, and prestige—now
all he can think about is what lies within him:

> And his breath began to fail him all the worse because of his
> apprehension. Pakhom ran—his shirt and drawers clung to his
> body by reason of sweat—his mouth was parched. In his breast a
> pair of blacksmith's bellows, as it were, were working; and in his
> heart a mill was beating; and his legs were almost breaking down
> under him.

Like those of Frida Kahlo and James Joyce, Tolstoy's anatomic
metaphors are simple substitution metaphors, in which one object
(the lungs, the heart) is replaced by another (a pair of bellows, a
mill). In order to convey what is happening inside Pakhom's body,
Tolstoy draws on things that are easy to observe and understand.
Similarly, Kahlo's damaged spinal cord (and the pain that arises from
it) becomes a Greek column in ruins, requiring the support of a
sturdy brace to hold it up.

These substitution metaphors are particularly effective at representing physical sensations. The abrupt transfer of metaphor parallels
the abrupt shift of perspective that occurs in the consciousness of the
sufferer. Pain thrusts Kahlo, Dedalus, and Pakhom inward and away
from the world, forcing them to confront the voice of their bodies,
which demands to be heard. Typically that voice is difficult to understand and articulate unless it can be linked to familiar objects that are
more accessible: Greek columns, faucets, bellows, and mills. The fact
that the substitutions are artifacts is especially suggestive. Like many

mechanical objects, the body requires a great deal of effort to keep it going: just as the blacksmith must work harder to heave his bellows more rapidly, so must the lungs work harder to take in more oxygen. Also like such objects, the body has inherent limitations, its own mortality: the bellows will eventually stop working, as might the lungs; the column will eventually collapse, as might the spine, which would lead to a literal breaking down of the person. Clearly, these metaphors compel us to see the body in an insightful way that would not have been accomplished by using literal words.

Another instance where an artifact is transported into the human interior to underscore its frailty occurs in Charles Dickens's *Bleak House*. During the course of the novel we encounter a homeless boy in the final stages of tuberculosis. Jo is ragged and shaking; his face is hollowed out, and he has an emaciated glare. But Jo's biggest problem is that he can no longer breathe effortlessly. He must expend considerable energy taking in and letting out air. The difficult breathing interferes with his ability to talk. Dr. Woodcourt encourages him, saying, "Draw breath, Jo."

"It draws," says Jo, "as heavy as a cart." He might add, "and rattles like it"; but he only mutters, "I'm a-moving on sir."

In a later conversation, it is obvious that talking and breathing are becoming increasingly difficult:

To Mr. Jarndyce, Jo repeats in substance what he said in the morning; without any material variation. Only, that cart of his is heavier to draw, and draws with a hollower sound.

Eventually the boy cannot muster enough strength to expand his constricted lungs:

For the cart so hard to draw, is near its journey's end, and drags over stony ground. All round the clock it labours up the broken steps, shattered and worn. Not many times can the sun rise, and behold it still upon its weary road. . . . The cart is shaken all to pieces, and the rugged road is very near its end.

Dickens's metaphor poignantly captures how his character feels when his lungs begin to fail; by transporting the cart into Jo's chest, the reader can visualize the body and its exhausting efforts to stay alive. The metaphor is particularly suited for a poor urban nomad, destined to roam from place to place until he can no longer do so. Even as he prepares to die, Jo and cart trudge on: "I'm a-moving on to the berryin ground—that's the move as I'm up to."

Jack London employs anatomic metaphor for similar effect in "Love of Life." A Yukon adventurer has sprained his ankle. After being abandoned by his only companion, he must travel alone and without food. Desperately trying to continue his journey, the man struggles to dismiss the worsening pain in his foot, since when he concentrates exclusively on the body, he becomes distracted and takes "no heed of the course he pursued." Only by ignoring the body's concerns can the man operate calmly and attend to his most pressing goal, survival. London, however, makes sure that we are aware of the man's pain at all times:

He groaned aloud as he started to drag himself to his feet. It was a slow and arduous task. His joints were like rusty hinges. They worked harshly in their sockets, with much friction, and each bending or unbending was accomplished only through a sheer exertion of will. When he finally gained his feet, another minute or so was consumed in straightening up, so that he could stand erect as a man should stand.

The metaphor draws an analogy between the human joint and the hinge. The substitution is effective, again, because the figurative image is accessible and because it evokes in sensuous detail the quality of pain experienced. The reader can see the slow, difficult movement of the rusty hinge and hear the grinding noises that are now occurring inside the sufferer. Only by understanding the man's pain, by sharing what he feels (albeit from a distance), is it possible for us to appreciate the man's tremendous will to survive, his love of life, as he momentarily defers the cries of the body and struggles on.

Like all the metaphors discussed in this book, anatomic metaphors work for both the sufferer and outside observers. Indeed, they bridge the divide between the two parties opened up by pain, making the experience more intelligible and more communicable at the same time. When scientists try to make sense of how the body (or the world) operates on a more objective level, they use them for the same purpose.

> The subjective experience of the body is usually incoherent and perplexing, and when we want to put it right, we refer to people who have learnt to think about it with the help of technical metaphors; experts whose use of analogy has enabled them to visualize the body not merely as an intelligible system but as an organized system of systems. . . . And since finding out what something is is largely a matter of discovering what it is like, the most impressive contribution to the growth of intelligibility has been made by the application of suggestive metaphors.

As Jonathan Miller points out, metaphors much like Tolstoy's and London's have played a prominent role throughout the history of science, from William Harvey's day (talking about the heart in terms of a pump) to the present (talking about the mind in terms of a computer.)

Yet most theorists of metaphor view simple substitution metaphors skeptically and are reluctant to ascribe to them the cognitive reach of more complex metaphors. The distinction is said to rest on grammatical structure. Substitution metaphors involve the *replacement of words* that have a secure and definite place in our vocabulary (heart for pump, hinge for joint). This type of metaphor, the argument goes, generates little conflict and can be easily paraphrased and interpreted. Interaction metaphor, the more complex species, involves a *transfer of terms at the level of the sentence*—as in Auden's poem "September 1, 1939": "The unmentionable odour of death / Offends the September night." Here there is as much tension between the terms—forebodings of war and an offending odor—as there is resemblance, both of which contribute to the metaphor's suggestiveness. Thus while lowly substitution metaphor is primarily decorative, according to Aristotle and Quintilian, interaction metaphor has the potential to formulate new categories and thereby add to our knowledge of the world, as per I. A. Richards, Max Black, Paul Ricoeur, and Nelson Goodman.

If we subscribe to this view, the substitution metaphors used by Kahlo, Tolstoy, and London become less impressive, their suggestiveness relatively constrained. But is that really true? We cannot easily paraphrase and interpret the metaphors by reversing the metaphorical transfer. Replacing Kahlo's column with an actual spine or changing Tolstoy's words to read "in his breast, the lungs were beating" would surely detract from the metaphors' added levels of meaning. The reclassification of body parts as artifacts makes us think of them in a novel way. So how can we reconcile the apparent contradiction that simple substitution may not always be so simple, that it can in certain instances be as evocative and conceptually dynamic as the interactive variety of metaphor?

Clearly there is a spectrum of metaphor, with those that are more decorative at one end and those that are more substantive at the other. But the distinction has to do more with the representational nature of a metaphor's subject—how well we understand and can talk about that subject—than with grammatical structure (word substitution versus interaction). When we compare two entities that have a fixed place in our collective understanding and vocabulary, we get metaphors that are more decorative and transparently "poetic." But when we view an indeterminate entity through the frame of a more determinate one, the metaphor actually *extends* our knowledge and vocabulary; we now have a way of understanding and talking about something that we didn't have before.

Structurally, the metaphors we have been discussing involve a substitution of words—column in place of spine, hinge in place of joint. In modern day they have a limited degree of suggestivity, because the spine, joint, and heart are not unknown entities; most of us, from the layperson to the scientist, are familiar with them. But if we turn back the clock, we would have to agree with Miller's claim that these "simple" metaphors must once have had tremendous reach. When Harvey started thinking of the heart in terms of the pump in the sixteenth century, it led to a paradigm shift in human physiology. Centuries of ignorance about circulation, dating back to Galen, were soon irrelevant. By mapping the inadequately understood organ onto the more determinate coordinates of the pump, scientists were able to advance their understanding of the heart.

Yet even today, despite the fact that our simple metaphors have a worn and dated feel, they are still suggestive, though perhaps less in terms of biology than in terms of phenomenology. For as we have seen, these metaphors speak about the body not only in a technical sense but also in an experiential one. Kahlo's column and London's rusty hinge call attention to how the spine and joint work as much as they do to what the pain issuing from their damaged surfaces feels like. And our experiences of the body are as difficult to know and talk about today as they were yesterday and as they will be tomorrow. Because the metaphors provide a meaningful representation of such experience, they are fitting and effective in a novel way.

Ultimately, what gives metaphors their cognitive reach and makes them indispensable has less to do with grammar than with their ability to let us see, know, and speak of something we can't see, know, or speak of—what we referred to earlier as their catachretic function. Whether in science, art, or religion, such metaphors operate as speculative instruments. By joining disparate domains, they help us "notice what would otherwise be overlooked" and "see new connections." Although theorists have struggled to specify exactly what is involved in this kind of "noticing" and "seeing"—is it a metaphorical seeing or a more literal one?—Nelson Goodman points to metaphor's facility at classifying things, a facility that must be understood not as a passive sorting out of predetermined object groupings but as an inventive and creative enterprise that *determines* such groupings in the first place. "The application of a label (pictorial, verbal, etc.)," argues Goodman, "as often *effects* as it records a classification."

Metaphor by definition operates through the transfer of labels. And like other modes of representation, its goal is to organize the world around or within us. In the case of London's character, an attempt is made to represent the way a sprained ankle might feel. However, difficulties immediately arise. How does one classify something one cannot observe or manipulate, something one cannot fully understand? The rusty-hinge metaphor obviates these difficulties precisely because its vehicle is better understood. The hinge's appearance (visual, auditory, even tactile) and its composition and mechanics provide structure and organization for the felt experience of a sprained ankle. In representation, writes Goodman,

> the artist must make use of old habits when he wants to elicit novel objects and connections. If his picture is recognized as almost but not quite referring to the commonplace furniture of the everyday world, or if it calls for and yet resists assignment to a usual kind of picture, it may bring out neglected likenesses or differences, force unaccustomed associations, and in some measure remake our world. And if the point of the picture is not only successfully made but is also well-taken, if the realignments it directly and indirectly effects are interesting and important, the picture—like a crucial experiment—makes a genuine contribution to knowledge.

WORD PICTURE: COMPLEX

We turn to several examples of more transparently suggestive metaphors used by people in pain. Structurally, they correspond to the interaction variety because they work in a more sustained manner throughout the sentences and paragraphs in which they appear. In addition, it would be difficult to say what the metaphors replace; paraphrasing them accurately becomes problematic, if not impossible. In these cases a sufferer, despite the lack of a literal discourse to represent his experience, looks metaphorically inside the body to see and now *describe* more systematically what is happening there—the layperson's version of what the philosopher Max Black calls the theoretical models found in science.

As she recounts in *Don't Leave Me This Way*, Julia Fox Garrison was thirty-seven years old when she suffered a massive brain hemorrhage that left her paralyzed. During the many months she spent in therapy following the stroke, Garrison couldn't stop thinking about the changes in her body. In the old days, she didn't have to think when she wanted to stand up or move around; she just stood up and moved at will.

> Your body's center of gravity is something you never gave much thought to before. The brain does many things unconsciously, things like breathing . . . and stabilizing itself when you lean forward to get a drink of water. The brain's the boss . . . supposedly. Currently though, some of your body parts are guilty of insubordination.

Post-stroke, however, Garrison has to consciously think about moving, just as Dickens's Jo has to consciously think about breathing; she is no longer detached from (and relieved of) the body's internal workings. But this doesn't necessarily allow her to move better, because as she discovers, there is now a disconnection between her brain and her limbs. To make sense of these facts, she envisions her body as a small business. The boss brain directs the worker limbs. Only the stroke has caused an insurrection in the workplace:

> In fact, the entire left side of your body now refuses to take orders from the boss. The boss is giving orders, but no one on the left side is listening. They've quit their jobs. So the boss has chosen to ignore the left side of your body. It no longer exists according to your brain.

The small business within her body (that is, the nervous system) led a relatively independent and autonomous existence before Garrison became ill. Now that the business is failing, the boss brain needs help from the owner Julia in order to get her worker limbs to move:

> My brain, which allowed me to be an independent human being for thirty-seven years or so, has decided to go on strike. I never had to think about each individual instruction the brain gives my limbs in order for me to walk or sit up erect in a chair. I'm not impulsive. I have never suffered from denial. My brain is just getting caught up to the fact that half of me is paralyzed and must be moved with conscious thought.

Although the metaphor might have been drawn out a little more clearly, it nonetheless provides Garrison with a useful picture. During rehabilitation therapy, she suffers physically as well as emotionally. Like all patients, she wants to know what happened to her and why. A partial explanation is obtained by envisioning the nervous system as a business. The metaphor exists in a space outside her, in words that her family and friends and readers of her story can also understand. In being able to convey how she feels, Garrison becomes less isolated.

Although Jack London worked in the realm of fiction rather than memoir, he suffered a great deal throughout his life and as a result became quite adept at conveying the pain of his imaginary characters. One of them, the unnamed man in his short story "To Build a Fire," does not survive his journey across the treacherous Yukon. Arrogant and unimaginative, the man doesn't appreciate the consequences a temperature of seventy degrees below zero might have on his body. He seems to challenge the cold with his "unprotected high cheekbones" and "his eager nose thrust aggressively into the air." But when he is unable to build a fire and starts to freeze, he can no longer ignore his body. London helps him and his readers understand what is happening in the man's interior through the use of anatomic metaphor.

As he struggles to keep warm, the man notices that his nose and cheeks become numb unless he rubs them with his mittens. Later on, he's not sure how he feels or if he even feels at all—whether his fingers are cold, painful, or simply senseless. It's only by violently flinging them against his chest that he recovers sensation. These observations are clarified when the man slips into a spring and is forced to stop and build a fire. Previously the exercise of walking was sufficient to warm his entire body. Once he stopped, "the pump eased down."

The blood of his body recoiled before it [the blow of the cold]. The blood was alive, like the dog, and like the dog it wanted to hide away and cover itself up from the fearful cold. So long as he walked four miles an hour, he pumped that blood, willy-nilly, to the surface; but now it ebbed away and sank down into the recesses of his body. The extremities were the first to feel its absence. His wet feet froze the faster, and his exposed fingers numbed the faster, though they had not yet begun to freeze. Nose and cheeks were already freezing, while the skin of all his body chilled as it lost its blood.

Unimaginative as he is, the man cannot fail to recognize and attempt to make sense of the cold's effects upon his body; his survival depends on it. Interestingly, he envisions "the blood" as a living, independent entity that he has little control over. Against his own wishes, the blood actively secures a place for itself in the warm recesses of his body and ignores his freezing extremities. It is only when he is active and moving that he can exert some pressure on the wayward organ; the pump (heart), energized, will reverse the selfish movement of the blood, propelling it in the opposite direction, outward toward the needy surfaces of the body.

The man's hypothetical model of the circulatory system does not correspond precisely to the scientific one. Although he has taken into account the raw data available to him, there is much that occurs below the threshold of his consciousness. In addition, the overall integration of and rationale for what happens in his body are beyond the scope of the man's education and imagination. He probably doesn't know the hierarchy of the organs involved, or that the brain is orchestrating events. Recognizing the drop in temperature, it directs the heart to slow down, the blood vessels at the periphery to constrict, and those in the core to dilate. The blood, with its heat-generating capacity, is thereby diverted away from the surface of the body and toward its interior. In this way, the more essential organs of the body—the heart, lungs, and brain—are maintained at the expense of the more expendable ones, the limbs.

The disparity between the scientist's and the layman's models is primarily one of scale. If London's man doesn't entirely understand the overall process, he has nevertheless put forth an intelligible and coherent account of how the body responds to dangerously low temperatures. He recognizes the fundamental role the circulatory system plays in these responses. He also appreciates his relative lack of control over the system. In his metaphor, the blood functions as a living organism within an organism. It hides like a dog in the nooks of his body to protect itself from the cold and in doing so ignores his hands and feet, their pain and subsequent destruction. Moreover, the metaphor is useful; it includes ways to modify the scripted responses. By flailing his hands, he can force the selfish blood back to the body's surface in order to feel his extremities again. Finally, the metaphor makes the man aware of the precariousness of his situation. He has made a grave mistake traveling alone in the Yukon at this time of year, just as the old-timer warned at the beginning of his journey.

Another, potentially more devastating effect of the cold occurs when the nervous system begins to fail, which evokes Julia Fox Garrison's experience after her stroke. The man's fingers, deprived of blood-borne oxygen, are not only numb or sense*less* but also unable to carry out his commands: "Lifeless they were, for he could scarcely make them move together to grip a twig, and they seemed remote from his body and from him." In order to move his hands, the man must, for the first time in his life, rely on additional sensory faculties to compensate for his absent sense of touch. He has to use his eyes ("When he touched a twig, he had to look and see whether or not he had hold of it") and his ears ("He knew the bark was there, and, though he could not feel it with his fingers, he could hear its crisp rustling as he fumbled for it") while he gropes awkwardly to build the fire that could save his life.

The man explains these phenomena by imagining the body as made up of a network of wires which connects the body's separate parts and facilitates communication between them. By damaging certain circuits in the network, the cold prevents the man from "talking" to his extremities. So when he can't feel his hands close on the twig, he decides that "the wires were pretty well down between him and his finger-ends." Later on, when he struggles to grip the matches and eventually has to give up, there can be only one explanation:

He watched, using the sense of vision in place of that of touch, and when he saw his fingers on each side of the bunch, he closed them—that is, he willed to close them, for the wires were down, and the fingers did not obey.

The network of wires is an ingenious way of representing the nervous system. It enables London's man to understand not only what happens when the system fails but also how it works in the healthy body. For the first time in his life, the man is functionally cut off from parts of his body that are still very much with him. He sees hands on the ends of his arms, but they don't seem to be his:

> He had an impression that they hung like weights on the ends of his arms, but when he tried to run the impression down, he could not find it.

The man comes to realize that even though the body remains intact, a sense of wholeness registers only when the network is fully operational and he is able to manipulate his body at will. In the terminology of neuroscience, the body's homunculus or self-image depends on a constant stream of incoming (sensory) and outgoing (motor) signals converging on the cortex.

While the nervous system is responsible for coordinating movement and assuring bodily integrity, the man also comes to appreciate its critical role in establishing contact with the external world. As Merleau-Ponty suggests, the healthy subject endlessly transcends himself (what he refers to as *ek-stase*) by rising toward the world with the body as intermediary. Through movement, speech, perception (all projects involving the body), we familiarize ourselves with the space we occupy in-the-world; we enter it and become part of it. "Our body is not in space like things," says Merleau-Ponty. "It inhabits or haunts space." When the wires break down, however, the range of possible motor projects narrows, thereby precipitously shrinking the space a person inhabits. We might say that London's man begins to lose his place in the world. When he attempts to stand, he must constantly observe his feet:

> He glanced down at first in order to assure himself that he was really standing up, for the absence of sensation in his feet left him unrelated to the earth.

The failure of the nervous system causes the man to lose contact with the rest of his body and with the world around him. Fittingly, he envisions himself as a winged Mercury "skimming along above the surface," unconnected to the earth.

The reference to the ancient god of communication underscores the central problem at the heart of London's text as well as many of the others encountered in this book—one that unfolds on three distinct levels. First, the sufferer is literally severed from the rest of the world by his environment, which must be traversed—that is, communicating at the macroscopic level—in order to reap the healing benefits of being reintegrated in society. At the same time, the sufferer is consumed by pain, which he urgently desires to understand and convey to others; thus, he is actively engaged in making his pain communicable. Finally, at the microscopic level and the ultimate source of his suffering, there is a breakdown in communication between the constituents of his body. In the case of London's man, the blood cells are prevented from delivering oxygen to the cells of the extremities, which begin to perish. By developing a crisis of communication on each of these levels, such stories are uniquely rewarding and helpful in trying to formulate a language of pain.

GOOD PAIN

There is another insight about pain, perhaps counterintuitive, to be gleaned from London's short story. Thus far we have talked about pain as a categorically negative experience. But as suggested earlier, we must be wary of any strictly monochromatic view, for pain comes in many different shades. It can be interpreted in different ways by people of different cultures and different times in history. Its meaning may even change for a particular person, depending on the context.

Like most people, London's man no doubt wanted to avoid pain at all costs before his fatal adventure. Yet as he freezes to death in the Yukon, he has a dramatic change of heart. Suddenly he sees pain in a positive light, embracing and even praying for its return. Though distressed that his fingers and nose hurt, the man is absolutely beside himself when the pain turns into numbness. He will do everything in his power, from running to shaking his hands, to experience those painful sensations again:

> After a time he was aware of the first faraway signals of sensation in his beaten fingers. The faint tingling grew stronger till it evolved into a stinging ache that was excruciating, but which the man hailed with satisfaction.

In this instance, pain actually *reassures* the man that his body is intact. When sensation returns, even for a brief moment, the isolated fragments of his body are reconnected; running properly, the network of wires makes the man whole again. As he comes to realize, that wholeness depends on a healthy nervous system, on a constant stream of incoming and outgoing signals registered in the brain.

Perhaps any sensation would be reassuring to the man at this moment, even an itch or a twinge. But pain is by far the *most* reassuring. As Elaine Scarry suggests, pain may exist as the primary model of certainty. It assures London's man not only that his body is whole but that it is still alive. When the hand has no pain, it ceases to exist. This most immediate, indubitable, and intense sensation is by these very qualities able to validate our existence. The German philosopher Martin Heidegger was sensitive to the paradoxical nature of pain, noting that it could be disruptive and constitutive simultaneously:

> But what is pain? Pain rends. It is the rift. But it does not tear apart into dispersive fragments. Pain indeed tears asunder, it separates, yet so that at the same time it draws everything to itself, gathers it to itself. Pain is the joining agent in the rending that divides and gathers. Pain is the joining of the rift.

The positive side of pain contributes to its survival value and derives from its connection to injury. Pain prompts us to withdraw our hand from the flame so that we prevent further damage to the body. It also prompts us to remember what has hurt us in the past so that we can be more careful in the future. Finally, it urges us to rest, allowing the body's "natural recuperative and disease-fighting mechanisms" to repair the damage.

But perhaps the most compelling evidence of pain's value is manifest when pain is absent, as it is for London's man, who does everything in his power to restore its presence. We also see this in medicine, in patients with diseases like leprosy and diabetes and in those born with varying degrees of pain insensitivity. When the nervous system is unable to provide the warning signal of pain, such patients injure themselves repeatedly. The injuries may lead to the loss of toes, fingers, and in some cases entire limbs, progressively fragmenting the body.

In the midst of suffering from a rare and painful disease called ankylosing spondylitis, the writer and editor Norman Cousins tried to reconcile these conflicting views of pain. How could someone in his right mind want what I am feeling at the moment? he wonders aloud in his memoir, *Anatomy of an Illness*. How could anyone possibly consider pain a good thing? And yet in certain instances it is without question good, even life-saving. Reflecting on Dr. Paul Brand's tireless efforts on behalf of leprosy patients in India, Cousins writes that if Brand were able, he would surely "move heaven and earth just to return the gift of pain to people who do not have it."

In a sense, the categorization of pain is as indeterminate as the sensation itself. It resists neat definitions and categorical statements. As the renowned pain physiologist Ronald Melzack freely admits, it remains a puzzle in many ways. There are times when pain is present without injury, when pain is disproportionate to the injury suffered, or when injury is present without any pain. What may be a "gift" to the leper or the diabetic is a nightmare to a person with a phantom limb, a brachial plexus injury, or migraine headaches. What may serve as a warning signal for the person about to step into the fire is a harbinger of death for the patient with metastatic cancer. The famous surgeon René Leriche once indignantly wrote:

> Physicians too readily claim that *pain is a reaction of defence, a fortunate warning, which puts us on our guard against the risks of disease*. . . . Reaction of defence? Against whom? Against what? Against the cancer which not infrequently gives little trouble until quite late? Against heart afflictions which always develop quietly? One must reject, then, this false conception of beneficent pain.

Regardless of the difficulties in rigidly categorizing the experience, however, there is no question that pain is the ultimate reality. While London's character desperately clings to that reality, others, like Norman Cousins, prefer that it never was.

THE WORLD IN PAIN

We turn now to a more indirect and subtle use of anatomic metaphors. In the following stories, writers spend a great deal of effort to create settings that mirror the felt experience of their characters' suffering. These "artifactualized" settings resemble projection metaphors, in which external objects—a boat, a tree, a piece of clothing—are remade to feel pain. Now, however, the same kinds of objects are appropriated as referents for what lies behind pain, for internal organs and systems that are damaged and failing. An example of this strategy in the visual arts is the fractured landscapes that appear in many of Frida Kahlo's paintings, including *Roots*, *The Broken Column*, and *Tree of Hope*—a *terra* that is no longer *firma* enough, like Kahlo's fractured spine, to be able support the weight of the human body. Here the external world not only is made to hurt like Frida (it feels pain) but also bears the same kind of hurt (the same kind of physical damage) present inside Frida's body.

This type of projection, in which the world reflects some aspect of humanity, is commonplace throughout the history of art and literature. The Romantic poets, for example, believed that our mental life, specifically the imagination and its artistic creations, is mirrored in

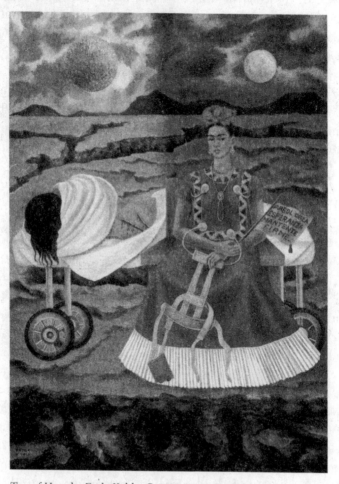

Tree of Hope by Frida Kahlo. © 2009 *Banco de Mexico Diego Rivera Frida Kahlo Museums Trust, Mexico, D.F. / Artists Rights Society (ARS).*

the organic origins, growth, and evolution of the natural world, in particular plants. According to the English poet and critic Samuel Coleridge, our ideas are "living and life-producing" and "essentially one with the germinal causes of nature." Contemporary theorists make humbler claims with their metaphorical projections. Instead of finding humanity in the larger world "out there," they find it in the smaller, self-contained world of the text. Moreover, the texts don't actually *refer* to human experience but rather *evoke* it. Poets use words and symbols—what T. S. Eliot called "objective correlatives"— to create a "mood" for their work that suggests and stirs up specific emotions in readers.

A fine example is the description of the outgoing tide at the beginning of Nellie Hermann's novel *The Cure for Grief*. In order to come to terms with the many losses she has suffered, Ruby Bronstein must first revisit them in turn. She must return to her childhood, to the private and distressing origins of her grief. Hermann's image of the ocean (the epigraph to this chapter) sweeping out and exposing its "muddy undersides and vulnerabilities" beautifully evokes her character's emotions at the outset of the novel: Ruby's desire to uncover meaning in the murky depths of memory and her anticipation of the fear, embarrassment, and pain that will accompany her journey.

Artists also regularly find the human body (as opposed to the mind) in the actual or textual world, especially the body's sexual aspects. The history of art is filled with symbols of male and female genitalia and representations of erotic desire and passion, from the Bronze Age figurines of Mother Earth and Sappho's poetry to the more recent work of D. H. Lawrence and Georgia O'Keeffe. In *Lady Chatterley's Lover*, Lawrence's metaphors enable his characters and readers both to see the sexual body from the outside and to see and feel it from the inside:

> To-day she could almost feel it in her own body, the huge heave of the sap in the massive trees, upwards, up, up to the bud-tips, there to push into little flamey oak-leaves, bronze as blood. It was like a

tide running turgid upward, and spreading on the sky. . . . She was gone in her own soft rapture, like a forest soughing with the dim, glad moan of spring, moving into bud. . . . She was like a forest, like the dark interlacing of the oakwood, humming inaudibly with myriad unfolding buds.

But while the erotic body has been well represented, the rest of the body (healthy or sick) has been much ignored. As Virginia Woolf pointed out, literature is more concerned with the mind. Even in many pathographies, narratives that have as their subject the sick body, we often hear more about the emotional than the physical aspects of the experience. Surely this has a lot to do with the body's inherent opacity and our tendency to "pass by it in silence" (Sartre). Even in illness and pain, when we're confined to the sickbed and can't ignore the welling up of the body—even then we continue to submerge and silence it.

Because of this absence, Frida Kahlo is unique in the history of art, while Tolstoy, London, and the many patients who have written so eloquently about their experiences in memoirs are unique in the history of literature. For these artists and ordinary people, the need to know and speak about the source of their pain is stronger than the obstacles preventing them. Instead of turning away, they fearlessly confront their bodies, painting and writing about how they feel and what they see. But while the subject matter of these works may be unique, the ways in which that subject matter is conveyed are not. The only way to represent internal experience—whether our emotions, sexuality, or pain—is to think and speak about it in terms of external objects.

Anton Chekhov's story "Gusev" revolves around a group of consumptives aboard a ship that will travel as far and as long as it takes for all of them to die. From the outset, we learn that the passengers have difficulty breathing. The heat and constant pitching of the boat exacerbate the problem:

[Pavel Ivanych] sleeps sitting up, as he cannot breathe lying down. . . . He is utterly worn out by his cough, by the stifling heat, his illness, and he breathes with difficulty, moving his parched lips.

Normally, respiration is an automatic process that slips back and forth along the border of consciousness. But when the lungs are damaged, in this case by tuberculosis, and respiration becomes increasingly difficult, it inevitably positions itself at center stage.

Chekhov himself suffered from tuberculosis and spent the last years of his short life in and out of sanatoriums. In order to convey the experience to his readers—his experience as well as his characters'—Chekhov must make us aware of the act of breathing. He does so by repeatedly juxtaposing descriptions of the ship (rolling and pitching) and the bunk (rising and falling) with descriptions of the ill men (inspiring and expiring). Common to each is a rhythm, at times monotonous and stable, at other times awkward and labored:

The ship is apparently beginning to roll. The bunk slowly rises and falls under Gusev as though it were breathing, and this occurs once, twice, three times.

Miming the movements of the sick body, the ship begins to breathe just like its occupants. As a result, the reader notices, even if only dimly, the rising and falling of the diaphragm that permits the exchange of oxygen and carbon dioxide to and from the body, the disruption of this vital rhythm, and the suffering that results when the process begins to fail.

In his novel *Our Mutual Friend*, Dickens represents the experience of the orphan Our Johnny in a similar way. Like Pavel Ivanych, Our Johnny struggles to breathe, probably because he too has tuberculosis. But where Chekhov sees the breathing process in the movement of a ship, Dickens sees it in the spinning of a wheel. In both cases the body is objectified, turned inside out so that other people can see and talk about it. Dickens's metaphor is so effective, its "reality" so transparent and credible, that it becomes difficult for both the sufferer and his caretakers to distinguish the "rattle-like" sounds and "lumbered" movements of the spinning wheel from those of Our Johnny's failing lungs:

> "Last night," said Sloppy, "when I was a-turning at the wheel pretty late, the mangle seemed to go like Our Johnny's breathing. It begun beautiful, then as it went out it shook a little and got unsteady, then as it took the turn to come home it had a rattle-like and lumbered a bit, then it come smooth, and so it went on till I scarce know'd which was mangle and which was Our Johnny. Nor Our Johnny, he scarce know'd either, for sometimes when the mangle lumbers he says, 'Me choking, Granny!' and Mrs. Higden holds him up in her lap and says to me 'Bide a bit, Sloppy,' and we all stops together. And when Our Johnny gets his breathing again, I turns again, and we all goes on together."

While Chekhov's and Dickens's metaphors focus on respiration, Max Brand, the pen name of Frederick Faust, who wrote in the early twentieth century, is concerned with representing the body's need for water in his short story "Wine on the Desert." Durante is a murderer trying to evade a posse chasing him through the desert. Along the way he stops at his friend Tony's house to refill his canteen. There, in the midst of an otherwise barren landscape, we encounter a remarkable sight: a thriving vineyard sustained by an elaborate system of interconnecting tanks and pipes, which collects and stores whatever scant rainwater falls. Durante takes what he needs and then riddles the water tanks with bullet holes so the posse won't be able to replenish its supplies. Ironically, though, Tony has replaced the water in Durante's canteen with wine, and Durante soon suffers an agonizing death in the desert.

How would it feel to die of thirst? We get a partial answer early on in the story, when Durante learns that Tony's father suffered this very fate. He asks Tony to elaborate:

"Did he just drop down and die?"

"No," said Tony. "When you die of thirst, you always die just one way. . . . First you tear up your shirt, then your undershirt. That's to be cooler. . . . And the sun comes and cooks your bare skin. . . . And then you think . . . there is water everywhere, if you dig down far enough. You begin to dig. The dust comes up through your nose. You start screaming."

As if this straightforward but circumstantial account is not entirely satisfactory, Brand then approaches the question in a more indirect fashion. Like Wittgenstein's interlocutor, Brand isn't content with a description of the sufferer's behavior. *That's what happens on the outside,* he might say, *a consequence but not the equivalent of how one feels inside.* Instead, Brand wants to know (and wants his reader to know) what is happening inside the body and how it feels.

Brand anatomizes the experience of water deprivation by setting up a series of polar images that represent the body replete with and bereft of water. In most cases the body is metaphorically displaced onto the natural elements and artifacts of the textual world. In this way Brand transforms the inaccessible realm of bodily sensation into the more accessible realm of perceptual experience. The basic question becomes less "What does it look like from the outside?" or even "How does it feel?"—which is understandably difficult to capture in language—than "What does it look and sound like from the inside?" The reader is made to see, hear, smell, and taste events occurring within the body.

In the first instance, when water is plentiful, the reader finds images of drinking and swallowing, of water permeating matter. We learn that Tony has planted his vines in a hollow. The lowness of the ground facilitates the movement of water into the tanks during the wet season:

The rains sank through the desert sand, through the gravels beneath and gathered in a bowl of clay hardpan far below.

This passive movement becomes a more active one when the land begins to drink the precious nutrient and make human sounds in the process:

> And the rain came down, and all the earth made a great hushing sound as it drank. Durante had heard the whisper of drinking when he was here before . . . the noise of the earth drinking was audible.

Just as the earth benefits from the nourishing properties of water, so too do man-made objects. Stone jars, whose surfaces resemble human skin, and the house take in whatever they can:

> There were two jars made of a porous stone, very ancient things, and the liquid which distilled through the pores kept the contents cool.

> It seemed to him that heat was radiating like light from his clothes, from his body, and the cool dimness of the house was soaking it up.

The metaphor is rounded out and completed when Durante drinks and feels the water "soaking through his body."

These images—of the earth, objects, and people drinking, of water moving through living and nonliving matter, of the sounds and scents that accompany it—suggest well-being, growth, and fertility. In the presence of water, the vines are healthy, displaying their large white blossoms with golden hearts "that poured sweetness on the air." In the presence of water, the vines are cool, just as Durante is when he plunges the dipper into the jar, "until the delicious coolness closed well above his wrist."

At the same time Brand creates an array of opposing images. Matter, no longer soaking up water, begins to wither and lose its material substance. The vines become wretched, dying things whose leaves hang "in ragged tatters." So too the tongue of the parched coyote that passes Durante in the desert:

> [It] hung out like a little red rag from the side of his mouth; and suddenly Durante was dry to the marrow.

Finally Brand transfers the image of the dry rag to the human body as Durante's tongue "cleaves to the roof of his mouth."

Deprived of water, the pores of material objects begin to fill up with a suffocating dust: Tony's patio, Durante's clothes, the vines, and then Durante himself. The air becomes stagnant and stale. Red becomes the dominant color as the sun, "a bowl of reddish soup," negates the cooling effects of water and reverses its previous flow.

> The sun struck through the east window and started them sweating . . . it turned the sweat of Durante into hot water and then dried his skin so that his clothes felt transparent.

The stars whirl into "little racing circles and scrawls of red." Then come the vultures, displaying their prominent red necks.

We are now ready for the final scene. Thanks to Brand's metaphors, the reader has been primed to understand what it may feel like to die of thirst. We see withered leaves, tongues that hang like rags, and an enveloping redness. We can smell and taste the alkaline dust. At the same time we remember the sight, feel, and sound of water permeating matter, just as Durante does when he becomes so debilitated that he mistakenly hears those exquisite sounds in "the swishing of the soft, deep sand through which he was treading." Unfortunately, the life-sustaining nutrient does not return until after Durante's death. Here again we are prepared for its reassuring voice:

Afterward, after many hours, out of the blind face of that sky the rain began to fall. It made first a whispering and then a delicate murmur like voices conversing, but after that, just at the dawn, it roared like the hoofs of ten thousand horses.

While Brand focuses primarily on what it feels like for a person to be with and without water, he is also concerned with how the body works to maintain a constant supply of this vital nutrient. Early on in the story, we encounter Tony's elaborate network of pipes and tanks, which collects, stores, and directs the flow of water to his vines:

In the middle of the rainless season, the well ran dry, but long before that, Tony had every drop of the water pumped up into a score of tanks made of cheap corrugated iron. Slender pipe lines carried the water from the tanks to the vines and from time to time let them sip enough life to keep them until the winter darkened overhead suddenly, one November day, and the rain came down, and all the earth made a great hushing noise as it drank.

Tony's network resembles the circulatory system. The heart (tanks) pumps blood (water) into slender vessels (pipes); in turn, the vessels transport the blood to the tissues of the body (vines). Certainly the network lacks the complexity and sophistication of the human body. Nevertheless, Brand's anatomic metaphor provides us with a concrete way of thinking and talking about one of the body's most critical systems and the consequences of its breakdown or removal of its supply of nourishment.

THE OUTSIDE IN THE INSIDE

Pain is difficult to express because it isn't necessarily connected to objects or referents in the shared, outer world. To overcome this obstacle, a person might imaginatively create a referent through metaphor. The material we have looked at during the course of this book, from the actual words of patients to works of fiction and art, offers three strategies for the creation of such referents. First, an agent in the outside world can be identified as acting against a person and causing pain. Next, the world can be remade to experience pain and empathize with a sufferer. And finally, the body can be opened up, enabling the sufferer to picture the internal source of pain. An overall structure for these strategies is the progressive interiorization of the experience. Pain is conceived as wholly external in the agency metaphor, as on the border between external and internal in the projection metaphor, and as wholly internal in the anatomic metaphor.

Yet while this sequence seems to move unidirectionally into the body, there is at the same time an unmistakable movement in the opposite direction, for when at last we arrive at the very core of the body, we find ourselves in the midst of the world beyond it. As we approach the heart, lungs, and joints, we encounter the pump, bellows, and hinge. Inasmuch as London's character moves further inside the body in an effort to understand the nervous system, he moves simultaneously outward into the external world when he discovers the network of wires. As a result, there is an obvious blurring of the categories initially and unambiguously labeled "inner" and "outer."

Nor should we be surprised that of all the worldly objects a person finds inside himself, the artifact is most conspicuous. These man-made objects, whether they are a series of words in a story or the objects these words signify, exist on the threshold between what lies within and what lies beyond the body. Projections of the human body and its sentience, they are at the same time tangible parts of the external world. For this reason, human artifice represents a node of continuity between our embodied selves and the world. Even more, it works to conflate the two by first externalizing (and objectifying) human sentience and then internalizing (and subjectifying) the world. In a compelling passage, Scarry reflects on this paradox of finding the "outside" in the "inside," the "public" within the "private," the "material" within the "spiritual"—all of which is brought about by acts of creation:

[The] very fact that a person looking straight forward at her physical image in the mirror or looking down at her own embodied circumference "sees" that she is "not just" and "much more than" a body . . . is itself at its origins a profound registration of the fact that physical sentience has, after first projecting itself outward, then absorbed back into its own interior content the externalized objectifications of itself. That is, human beings project their bodily powers and frailties into external objects such as telephones, chairs, gods, poems, medicine, institutions, and political forms, and then those objects in turn become the objects of perception that are taken back into the interior of human consciousness where they now reside as part of the mind or soul, and this revised conception of oneself—as a creature relatively untroubled by the problem of weight (chair), as one able to hear voices coming from the other side of the continent (telephone), as one who has direct access to an unlimited principle of creating (prayer)—is now actually "felt" to be located inside the boundaries of one's own skin where one is in immediate contact with an elaborate constellation of interior cultural fragments that seem to have displaced the dense molecules of physical matter. Behind the surface of the face in the mirror is blood and bone and tissue but also friends, cities, grandmothers, novels, gods, numbers, and jokes; and it is likely to be the second group (the socialization of sentience) rather than the first (the privacy of sentience) that she at that moment "senses" as the washcloth in the mirror moves back and forth over the illuminated surface of the skin.

Philosophers, at least since Descartes's time, have been troubled by the absolute divisions, ontological and epistemological, that appear to separate mind from body, inner from outer, and private from public. These divisions surface most dramatically in the setting of pain. Is pain a physical (bodily) or psychological (mental) event? Is it the most private and unknowable experience we have? And if so, are people in pain doomed to suffer alone and in silence like the figure in Munch's painting?

If there is a language of pain, how can we remain committed to such a pessimistic view? This is the rhetorical question Wittgenstein poses in his private-language argument. The vocabulary of the private world, he argues persuasively, cannot be detached from the public world. If it were, how could we ever teach our children the word "pain," use the word meaningfully, and understand others who use it? We can do all of these, so there must be a shared, public basis to the experience. That basis is the prelinguistic circumstances surrounding pain—the behavior of the sufferer, his expressions, the settings in which pain occurs, and the response of others. These circumstances provide a common foundation on which language can build.

This book has approached the same problem from a different perspective. Our point of departure was Wittgenstein's interlocutor, who remained dissatisfied with the philosopher's analysis and continued to insist that the only reality of his pain was inside him and private. We appeased the interlocutor, so to speak, by giving him permission to describe what his experience felt like "from the inside": since you must, tell us what you're pointing to, tell us what is going on in the privacy of your self. If the three metaphors regularly used by people in pain, real and fictional, are representative, the inner, private referents are as outer and public as the behavior Wittgenstein emphasizes. The language of agency, the projection of pain onto other objects, and the anatomic metaphors of the body's interior, whether formulated in pictures or in words, are unequivocally situated in the communal world.

It may be impossible to relinquish the notion that there exist within us realms of experience that remain strictly private and wholly our own. But the stinging Wittgensteinian rebuke remains: what do you actually have that you call your own which I cannot have and which lies beyond our shared language games? Even if we acknowledge the existence of such private experiences, we're compelled to say that they are as much or as little one's own as the multitude of bodily processes that occur below the threshold of awareness. And those that are felt are private inasmuch as they are elusive, indeterminate, and inaccessible. If we persist in granting a status to such categorically private experience, it can be in only the most insubstantial sense. Consciousness, Merleau-Ponty writes,

> does not begin to exist until it sets limits to an object, and even the phantoms of "internal experience" are possible only as things borrowed from external experience. Therefore, consciousness has no private life, and the only obstacle it encounters is chaos, which is nothing.

The private experience of pain resembles the private experience of thought, disintegrating as rapidly as it materializes. When we wish to pin it down, however, we must be able to express it:

> A thought limited to existing for itself, independently of the constraints of speech and communication, would no sooner appear than it would sink into the unconsciousness, which means that it would not even exist for itself.... [Thought] does indeed move forward with the instant and, as it were, in flashes, but we are then left to lay hands on it, and it is through expression that we make it our own.

Expression in this sense goes beyond communication. It is at the same time the apprehension of experience by providing it with a more lasting form and structure, by making it signify and mean something. And it is language above all that enables a person to detach experience from its elusive, private moorings and transform it into a meaning that can be shared. Our language can indeed represent our most intimate experiences, argues the philosopher Simon

Blackburn, as long as it relies on a public reality: "There is no 'private order,' any more than there is a private language to express it."

For these reasons, we must agree with Merleau-Ponty, Wittgenstein, Blackburn, and Scarry that there is no private order—human beings are in the world and know themselves in the world. As personal and subjective as pain appears, it must not be conceived as disconnected from the outside world. When, instead, we approach the experience like the real and fictional sufferers discussed in this book, as being receptive to language and meaning, its private and inner quality begins to dissolve. "Language leads us to a thought which is no longer ours alone, to a thought which is presumptively universal."

Postscript

> The limits of my language mean the limits of my world.
>
> —LUDWIG WITTGENSTEIN, *Tractatus*

> In my utopia, human solidarity . . . is to be achieved not by inquiry but by imagination, the imaginative ability to see strange people as fellow sufferers. . . . Solidarity is created by increasing our sensitivity to the particular details of the pain and humiliation of other, unfamiliar sorts of people . . . coming to see other human beings as "one of us" rather than as "them."
>
> —RICHARD RORTY, *Contingency, Irony, and Solidarity*

Is it really possible to express pain while we are experiencing it? And even if it is, how helpful would it be for us? Has there been a practical point to this exercise? Or has it been just another philosophical debate like the kind I used to have during graduate school at the local pub, which often rose to fever pitch and then quickly dissipated into the night air?

It's difficult to think of *the most eloquent expressions of pain* and *patients in the hospital* occupying the same breath. The lush metaphors of Joyce and Tolstoy seem so remote from the actual world of pain—a world that is barren and wordless. I have seen this in my career as a physician and also, more intimately, as a patient. Pain is all-consuming; it actively swallows up language as it does everything else. At its most intense, there is no time to think, let alone try to represent how one feels. Pain, as Munch's painting shows, silences us. So why bother trying to speak? Why not just close one's eyes, as I did many years ago in my hospital room, and wait for it to pass? And for those who witness pain, why bother trying to break down the wall of private experience and attempt to share what cannot be shared?

The simple answer is that we must. We must because the consequences of not trying are too great. As a practical matter, we need language to alleviate pain. Physicians rely on the stories of patients—how well they communicate their symptoms—as much as they do on stethoscopes and blood tests and imaging studies. The stories help them pinpoint the source of pain and prescribe appropriate medicine. When language is lacking, it becomes increasingly difficult for them to do their job and much more likely that pain will not be adequately treated.

But the consequences of not being able to express pain go beyond medicine, for pain, as we have seen, goes beyond medicine. Pain is present not only in psychiatric conditions such as depression but in the very midst of health, in the loss of a loved one, for example, or during times of extreme anxiety. Pain is not an aberration in human experience but a routine, inescapable part of life, as the Buddhists rightly recognize. It affects us all at one point or another. How, then, can we let it pass without trying to share it? How can we keep silent? Without language or some other form of representation, pain loses its substance and eventually ceases to exist. It becomes as abstract as the ideas debated over lagers at the pub and just as easy to turn and walk away from after last call—like the faraway suffering of children in Sudan and Malawi or the less remote suffering of cancer patients here in the United States, whose pain often goes unrelieved. It becomes in essence a *not-part* of everyday life that can easily be ignored and in some cases even dismissed.

Finally, the drying up of language is not merely a symptom but an ongoing source of pain. Undoubtedly there are many varieties of pain, each of which has its own particular characteristics; the pain from a broken leg may be qualitatively different from the pain of grief. Yet despite these differences, pain has a common underlying structure. No matter what the cause, it systematically destroys everything except itself and thereby isolates us from the world of family and friends and doctors. Language is a means to reverse this epoché, a bridge that can lead us directly back to the communal world. It is not only helpful to a physician in choosing the right medicine, it is *in itself a form of medicine*. Conversely, when language is absent, we feel even more isolated—an absence that inevitably exacerbates our pain, exacerbates what Styron referred to as the "aching solitude" of pain.

As inexpressible as pain seems, therefore, we cannot close our eyes and turn away. We must try to speak. Maybe not in every instance—when pain is at its worst—but later on, when it has subsided. Of course, as Daudet remarked, there is a certain artificiality and untruthfulness in talking "when everything is over." Language, it is true, comes after experience. It is like the subtitle of Crane's story—"A Tale intended to be after the Fact"—a postscript. But regardless of when it comes, language will always have value, because it can represent and validate this fundamental aspect of lived existence, because it can help physicians relieve pain, and because it is itself therapeutic.

What appears impossible is not impossible. Despite the problematic nature of pain—that it is inside us and private, that it is objectless and without form, and that it is inherently opaque—it remains open to language and can be meaningfully talked about. While pain threatens to destroy language, it doesn't always do so. Indeed, I have tried to show that a rhetoric of pain actually exists, one that can assume many shapes and forms, at times relatively commonplace and at others more imaginative and distinctive. While the language of agency is readily recognizable in everyday speech, the projection and anatomic metaphors of Tolstoy, London, Joyce, and Morrison are more transparently literary. We don't typically find people in the hospital sympathizing with the suffering of trees or talking about their earaches in terms of the roar of a train passing through a tunnel.

This, not surprisingly, brings up that nagging sense of impracticality all over again. What good are the solutions to the problem if they come from unusable sources? What good are Joyce's fanciful metaphors to the man in the street, to the person in the grip of pain? Questions like these are what drove me away from an academic career in literature and into the more practical realm of medicine. I decided that reading and writing about people who suffered wouldn't be fulfilling enough for me; I needed to do something about it.

But I no longer see things in black-and-white. I realize now that there is a profoundly practical side to literature, a side that is nowhere more evident than in the setting of pain. Pain challenges us, and challenges language, like no other experience we have. Because of its problematic nature, we can't express pain directly or literally; we can't point to it like we point to a bird in the sky and describe its features. The only way to talk of pain is indirectly or metaphorically. Right up front, we need to be more imaginative and creative than usual. We need to think more literarily. If we really want to convey how it feels, we need to think like Joyce and Tolstoy.

Moreover, since language is a dynamic and fluid activity, we need to continue thinking of pain like our best writers and continue creating novel ways to express it. Metaphors inevitably age and become part of literal discourse. Like antibiotics, they develop resistance, which deprives them of their descriptive and suggestive powers. To say that you have a splitting headache may not be enough anymore; the phrase has become so banal that it may not make us really *see* pain. And if we don't see it, then we can't know or talk about it very effectively, and others may be less likely to believe it. So we must continually revive our older metaphors, replace stabbing pain with more exotic versions of agency. And, equally important, we must come up with brand-new metaphors. Only we can't expect to find the next generation of metaphors in the pipelines of giant pharmaceutical companies like Pfizer and Johnson & Johnson. They will turn up instead in the works of our best writers and artists.

In his recent novel *The Yiddish Policemen's Union*, the Pulitzer Prize–winning author Michael Chabon is particularly adept at fashioning evocative metaphors to describe the felt experiences of his characters:

> Litvak stood up slowly, with a grunt of pain. There were screws in his hips, which ached; his knees thudded and gonged like the pedals of an old piano. There was a constant thrum of wire in the hinges of his jaw. He ran his tongue across the empty zones of his mouth with their feel of slick putty. He was accustomed to pain and breakage.

Chabon's anatomic metaphors bring the interior, subjective experience of pain out into the open. We can see, hear, and touch it. There is no possibility of closing our eyes and turning away, of not prescribing enough pain medication if Litvak walks into our emergency room.

Writers and artists teach us how to approach difficult-to-approach entities like pain. They teach us that if the interior world is less accessible than the exterior one, we need to remake that world so it becomes more accessible. We need to find external objects that can stand in for and refer to how we feel inside—objects like weapons and agents, for example, that threaten to injure our bodies; objects like the trees Vasili encounters in the snowstorm and other patients on our hospital ward that suffer in the same way we do; and objects "inside" us, like sinks and screws and old pianos that might serve as a source for our aversive sensations. These objects are eminently more describable than our vague interior experiences. As such, they make it possible to convey those experiences to others and more likely that others will respond in appropriate ways.

I don't mean to suggest that we can all write like the best novelists, let alone talk in the carefully considered manner in which they craft their stories. But at least we know how it might be done and that it can be done. The point is not necessarily to mime the words of Chabon or Tolstoy but to glimpse the range of the possible, to be aware of the ideal shape words might take, for that ideal then belongs to all of us. More than just communicating one person's experience, the metaphors of great writers contribute to our collective experience of pain. They add to our ever-growing repository of language and to our ever-growing understanding of what it means to be human. Indeed, we should think of our great artists no differently than our great scientists. Both have profoundly practical goals; each works to help us understand and talk about what is not fully understood or communicable. But where the scientist shines his searchlight on the objective world, the artist strives to illuminate the subjective one.

Above all, these writers make us appreciate the incredible power of language, especially in places inherently inhospitable to language. Just think of the characters in Tolstoy and London who find themselves in the desolate landscapes of the Russian steppes and the Yukon. Or of William Styron standing at the edge of depression's precipice—these moments of extremity, these reenactments of the felt experience of pain. Then think of the overwhelming desire and need to speak out in such instances, regardless of what emerges and how articulate it sounds. The human voice promises what may at times be the only escape from pain's epoché, the only way those in pain can preserve their dwindling connection to humanity—a matter of life and death. As Elaine Scarry says of three famous sufferers in literature, Oedipus, Lear, and Beckett's Winnie,

> Their ceaseless talk articulates their unspoken understanding that only in silence do the edges of the self become coterminous with the edges of the body it will die with.

Despite the challenge of pain, we cannot let it silence us. At the very least, we must make the attempt to speak, regardless of when that becomes possible—in the moment of pain or days, months, or even years later—and no matter what form or quality that speaking takes, whether it is a publishable book like Styron's or an informal posting on an Internet chat room. Language can alleviate pain. As long as the conversation lasts, writes the philosopher Richard Rorty, we remain unalterably embedded in a community of other human beings who may share our experience. As long as the conversation lasts, we are not alone.

Notes

Introduction

13   *"a state anterior to language"*: Scarry, *Body in Pain*, 4.

14   *"has an Element of Blank"*: Dickinson, poem 650 in *Complete Poems*, 323. All subsequent quotations from this poem are taken from this edition.

14   *"It is not talk"*: Auden, "Surgical Ward," in *Selected Poems*, 73. All subsequent quotations from this poem are taken from this edition.

14   *"Let a sufferer try"*: Woolf, "On Being Ill," 194.

14   *one out of every five Americans*: In its primary educational publication, the American Pain Society asserts that "about 9 in 10 Americans regularly suffer from pain, and pain is the most common reason individuals seek health care. Each year an estimated 25 million Americans experience acute pain due to injury or surgery and another 50 million suffer from chronic pain. Chronic pain is the most common cause of long-term disability, and almost one third of all Americans will experience severe chronic pain at some point in their lives." American Pain Society, *Pain*, 3.

16   *language of agency*: Scarry, *Body in Pain*, 15–19.

18   *"[There is] no general theory"*: Daudet, *In the Land of Pain*, 15.

20   *"Words only come"*: Ibid.

Chapter 1: The Quintessential Private Experience

24   *"He had just felt death"*: Hemingway, "The Snows of Kilimanjaro," 461.

25   *existence as a* being-in-the-world: During the course of this book, I draw on several phenomenological concepts (e.g., being-in-the-world, intentionality, and epoché) as they are used primarily in the work of Maurice Merleau-Ponty.

26   *"It is because we are through and through"*: Merleau-Ponty, *Phenomenology of Perception*, xiii.

27 *"But the harmonious, exemplary Rusanov family"*: Solzhenitsyn, *Cancer Ward*, 15.

28 *"How the world has changed"*: Woolf, "On Being Ill," 195.

28 *"almost sadder than death"*: Sacks, *A Leg to Stand On*, 65.

29 *"ferocious inwardness"*: Styron, *Darkness Visible*, 19–20.

30 *"fable-like days"*: Greenberg, *Hurry Down Sunshine*, 23–24.

31 *"imagine a form of torment"*: Styron, *Darkness Visible*, 17.

31 *"Romain told me"*: Ibid., 25–26.

32 *some deep subterranean fact*: Scarry, *Body in Pain*, 3.

33 *"For the person whose pain"*: Ibid., 4.

34 *researchers began to investigate*: See Marks and Sacher, "Undertreatment of Medical Inpatients."

35 *They had their reasons*: Patients are at times also responsible for the undertreatment of their pain. While physicians have their reasons for not prescribing adequate medication, patients have their reasons for not asking for or refusing medication. On occasion these reasons may overlap and be equally misguided (as in the fear of addiction).

35 *decades later, nothing had changed*: See U.S. Department of Health and Human Resources, *Management of Cancer Pain*. The undertreatment of pain in cancer patients has also been reported in England (Mayor, "Survey of Patients") and extends to patients with other conditions, including AIDS (Larue et al., "Underestimation and Undertreatment").

Chapter 2: The Elusiveness of Pain

38 *simply "indescribable"*: Styron, *Darkness Visible*, 16.

38 *"that 'having pain' may come"*: Scarry, *Body in Pain*, 4.

38 *"so incontestably and unnegotiably present"*: Ibid.

39 *"The merest schoolgirl"*: Woolf, "On Being Ill," 194.

39 *Pain, however, defies*: See Sartre, *Being and Nothingness*, 332–33; Trigg, *Pain and Emotion*, 5–20; Rorty, *Philosophy and the Mirror of Nature*, 22–24; and Scarry, *Body in Pain*, 161–62. There is, however, at least one philosopher who would disagree. Michael Tye believes that all feelings and experiences, even pain, have intentional content. In his view, pain is a sensory (and nonconceptual) *representation* of a bodily disturbance.

See *Ten Problems of Consciousness,* 93–131.) Still, I'm sure Tye would agree that those "bodily disturbances" are much more indeterminate (and therefore more difficult to express) than the intentional objects of most other inner experiences.

40   *intentionality is critical*: If we wish to represent consciousness, according to the philosopher Roderick Chisholm, we must mirror its intentional movements by using intentional language. See "Sentences about Believing," 124, and *Perceiving,* 172–73.

40   "*Yet it cannot be*": Freud, "Inhibitions, Symptoms and Anxiety," 171. See also pp. 131, 169.

41   "*The complex of melancholia*": Freud, "Mourning and Melancholia," 253. See also p. 244. Freud's insight is corroborated by the clinical overlap between psychological and physical pain. Depressed patients commonly exhibit somatic complaints while patients with physical illness often experience depression (especially those with chronic illness and intense physical pain).

42   "*three-quarters of badly wounded men*": Beecher, "Pain in Men Wounded in Battle," 99.

43   "*variable connection*": Melzack and Wall, *Challenge of Pain,* 3. See also Hampton, "A World of Pain," 2425–27.

44   *language, thought, politics*: See Johnson, *Body in the Mind,* 65–100.

45   *two fundamental modes of acquiring knowledge*: For the importance of perception to knowledge acquisition, see Merleau-Ponty, *Primacy of Perception,* 25, and Foucault, *Birth of the Clinic,* 114. For the importance of the judgment of others, see McGinn, *Wittgenstein on Meaning,* 48–92, and Rorty, *Philosophy and the Mirror of Nature,* 171ff. ("We understand knowledge when we understand the social justification of belief").

45   *the minor sensory organs*: For more on the indeterminacy of internal sensory experience, see Armstrong, *Bodily Sensations,* 33–35; Medvei, *Mental and Physical Effects of Pain,* 7; and Miller, *Body in Question,* 27.

46   "*No experience demands*": Bakan, *Disease, Pain, and Sacrifice,* 57–58. Pain is not unique, then, in lacking intentionality, since all internal sensations (twinges, aches, itches) share this characteristic. See Wittgenstein, *Blue and Brown Books,* 22, and Searle, *Intentionality,* 1. What sets pain apart is the distress this lack of intentionality causes us and the urgent need we feel to address it.

Chapter 3: The Public Side of Pain

50   "*Just try in a real case*": Wittgenstein, *Philosophical Investigations*, section 303.

52   *impossible to guarantee*: For more on the public criteria or rules of language, see Kripke, *Wittgenstein on Rules*, 3, 79, 89; Malcolm, *Nothing Is Hidden*, chap. 9; Hacker and Baker, *Scepticism, Rules and Meaning*, 42ff.; and McGinn, *Wittgenstein on Meaning*, 48–92.

52   "*Why can't my right hand*": Wittgenstein, *Philosophical Investigations*, section 268.

53   *Language, we come to realize*: For more on Wittgenstein's dynamic theory of meaning, where the meaning of a word is its use in the language, see Pitcher, *Philosophy of Wittgenstein*, 228–54; Bolton, *An Approach to Wittgenstein's Philosophy*, 109–19, 151–56; and Hacker, *Insight and Illusion*, 152.

53   "*In what sense have you got*": Wittgenstein, *Philosophical Investigations*, section 398.

54   "*Man is in the world*": Merleau-Ponty, *Phenomenology of Perception*, xi.

Chapter 4: Man's Puny Inexhaustible Voice

57   This, *insists the interlocutor*: Wittgenstein, *Philosophical Investigations*, sections 296, 298.

58   *the majority of people don't submit*: Frankl, *Man's Search for Meaning*, 54–108.

58   "*in order to live*": Didion, *White Album*, 11.

59   "*Nor can we know*": Didion, *Year of Magical Thinking*, 189.

59   "*No man is an island*": Donne, *Devotions upon Emergent Occasions*, 103.

60   "*thirsts for speech*": Chekhov, "Heartache," 124.

Chapter 5: Metaphor and Worldmaking

66   "*The white look*": Joyce, *Portrait of the Artist*, 250.

66   "*He leaned his elbows*": Ibid., 252.

67   "*The depressed person*": Wallace, "The Depressed Person," 57.

71   *Most theorists of metaphor*: See Aristotle, *Poetics*, 2332–33; Ricoeur, *Rule of Metaphor*, 22; and Goodman, *Languages of Art*, 72–74. Not surprisingly,

Derrida is quick to point out the circularity of defining metaphor with metaphor—for the notion of deviance, the *movement* from a home realm to an alien one, is blatantly metaphorical ("White Mythology," 28).

71   *"bump on the head"*: Davidson, "What Metaphors Mean," 44.

72   *our so-called literal language is saturated*: See Johnson and Lakoff, *Metaphors We Live By*. Max Black writes that considering its ubiquity in ordinary language, metaphor should seem "no more mysterious than singing or dancing—and, one might add, no more improper or deviant" ("More about Metaphor," 21).

72   *They behave like literary language*: For more on the estranging or defamiliarizing effects of art (*ostranenie* to the Russian formalists), see Shklovsky, "Art as Technique."

73   *According to Aristotle*: Aristotle, *Poetics*, 2250.

73   *language is inextricably entwined*: For more on the modern view of language that began with the comparative linguistic studies of Benjamin Whorf and Edward Sapir, see Henle, "Language, Thought, and Culture," and Pinker, *Stuff of Thought*, chap. 3, who calls attention to the different versions of the modern view. As an advocate of conceptual semantics, for example, Pinker argues that language is a window into human thought but doesn't actually determine the kinds of thoughts we can think (linguistic determinism).

74   *nominalism (of single words)*: See Ricoeur, *Rule of Metaphor*, 101–33.

74   *"The thing in the box"*: Wittgenstein, *Philosophical Investigations*, section 293.

75   *filling these voids*: See Soskice, who, unlike most theorists, emphasizes the singular nature of metaphor's subject rather than the interaction between two subjects (*Metaphor and Religious Thought*, 47–53).

75   *Only indirectly and figuratively*: Maimonides, *Guide for the Perplexed*, 11, 123, 133.

76   *But how do scientists conceptualize*: See Black, *Models and Metaphors*, 221–29, and Quine, "A Postscript on Metaphor," 159.

76   *In fact, the truth value*: Instead of truth value, Goodman talks about "rightness of fit" (*Ways of Worldmaking*, 17–22, and 129–39). On the other hand, Hesse (*Models and Analogies*, 162) and Boyd ("Metaphor and Theory Change," 357–68) want to affirm the truth value of scientific metaphor and therefore argue that it can refer to an entity determinately while representing it indeterminately. In this way, such metaphor

acts as a "guide" (Hesse) or an "invitation for further exploration" (Boyd), which can be revised over time as "it accommodates language to the causal structure of the world" (Boyd).

77 *We reach for it*: See Cassirer, *Language and Myth*, 83–99; Langer, *Philosophy in a New Key*, 26–52; and Rorty, *Contingency, Irony, and Solidarity*, 9–19.

78 *primordial existence*: Merleau-Ponty, *Phenomenology of Perception*, xi.

Chapter 6: The Weapon

82 *"utterly speechless"*: Burney, *A Known Scribbler*, 303.

83 *"Strange aches; great flames"*: Daudet, *In the Land of Pain*, 6, 21.

83 *"The anesthesia wore off"*: Price, *Whole New Life*, 26.

84 *"This lethal eel"*: Ibid., 29.

84 *"Suddenly, two great claws"*: Hsi, *Closing the Chart*, 12.

85 *heavily armed conflict*: Donne, *Devotions upon Emergent Occasions*, 117–18.

86 *"No. I say No. Mr. Dubedat"*: Shaw, *Doctor's Dilemma*, 155–56.

86 *For Susan Sontag*: Sontag, *Illness as Metaphor*, 63–64.

87 *medical "smart bomb"*: See, for example, Michael Lasalandra, "Study: Smart Bomb Drug Targets Cancer," *Boston Herald*, May 21, 2002.

87 *"a war against cancer"*: Radner, *It's Always Something*, 124.

87 *"The secondaries were tearing"*: Solzhenitsyn, *Cancer Ward*, 58.

87 *can have harmful consequences*: Sontag, *Illness as Metaphor*, 42–48, 57–58.

89 *There are only two possibilities*: Wittgenstein, *Philosophical Investigations*, section 244. Wittgenstein is more concerned with rejecting what should *not* form the basis of a language of pain (private feelings) than with explaining what should (contexts and behaviors). Some of his followers went on to develop these latter themes more systematically, in particular David Pears in *False Prison*, 398–401.

89 *"primitive" and "prelinguistic"*: See Wittgenstein, *Zettel*, section 541, and *Remarks on the Philosophy of Psychology*, vol. 1, section 916.

92 *difficult to categorize pain*: See Sternbach, *Pain*, 11, and Melzack and Wall, *Challenge of Pain*, 15–33.

92   "a pure physical experience": Scarry, Body in Pain, 52.

96   "Pain is the unpleasant sensory": International Association for the Study of Pain, "Pain Terms," 249.

96   "terrible wounds": Jamison, Unquiet Mind, 39.

96   The dense thicket of scar tissue: Morrison, Beloved, 18 (see also pp. 20, 93, 109).

Chapter 7: Literary Agency

98   "is to make the felt tensions": S. Langer, Mind, 51.

99   London, we know: See "Introduction," in Short Stories of Jack London, xix, xxx.

100 "Nature has many tricks": London, "The White Silence," 10.

101 "forces its way": Tolstoy, "Lost on the Steppe," 178. All subsequent quotations from this story are taken from this edition.

102 "the marrow of her bones": Maupassant, "The First Snowfall," 253. All subsequent quotations from this story are taken from this edition.

103 Pain is a warning signal: In his book Feeling Pain and Being in Pain (7–40), Nikola Grahek persuasively shows that anticipation and threat are central to the experience of pain by discussing two rare syndromes in which the affective, cognitive, and behavioral components of pain are completely dissociated from the sensory component. In the case of pain asymbolia, when a patient has pain but is indifferent to it, pain "comes to nothing in the sense that it is no longer a signal of threat or damage for the subject, and doesn't move his mind or body in any way." For this and other reasons, Grahek believes that the basic representational and motivational force of pain is not in its sensory component but rather in its affective, cognitive, and behavioral ones.

104 the pain of being deformed: Grealy, Autobiography of a Face, 7, 186.

104 "suffocated" and "drowned": Styron, Darkness Visible, 17.

104 Kahlo paints the emotional pain: See Herrera, Frida, 188–90.

105 "an impending destruction of the person": Cassell, Nature of Suffering, 33.

106 "We were Siamese twins": Levertov, "Divorcing," in Freeing of the Dust, 66.

107 "bringing about a reversion": Scarry, Body in Pain, 4.

109 *"None of them knew the color"*: Crane, "The Open Boat," 68. All subsequent quotations from this story are taken from this edition.

111 *an imaginative schema*: Johnson, *Body in the Mind*, xix–xx, 42–48.

111 *"The Argentine air force"*: Ibid., 89.

112 *"registering in its own contours"*: Scarry, "Introduction," xi.

112 *"The wind grew more violent"*: Hardy, *Woodlanders*, 285.

113 *"Sometimes a bough"*: Ibid., 285–86.

113 *"No; it is beyond me"*: London, "The Heathen," 378. All subsequent quotations from this story are taken from this edition.

115 *"The wind was no longer"*: London, "The House of Mapui," 319. All subsequent quotations from this story are taken from this edition.

116 *"The cold of space"*: London, "To Build a Fire," 288.

118 *"The habit of poets"*: Scarry, *Body in Pain*, 286.

119 *"that we can understand"*: Johnson and Lakoff, *Metaphors We Live By*, 34.

120 *"The wind stood up"*: Stephens, "The Wind," 268.

123 *Sontag rails against*: Sontag, *Illness as Metaphor*, 42–48, 57–58.

123 *"I shall know why"*: Dickinson, poem 193 in *Complete Poems*, 91.

124 *"to transform interior content"*: de Man, *Allegories of Reading*, 47.

125 *"We have learnt"*: Nietzsche, *Will to Power*, 9–10.

126 *"A* picture *held us captive"*: Wittgenstein, *Philosophical Investigations*, section 115.

126 *"only safely use"*: Wittgenstein, *Wittgenstein's Lectures*, 25.

Chapter 8: The Mirror

130 *"Don't be silly"*: Hemingway, "The Snows of Kilimanjaro," 444. All subsequent quotations from this story are taken from this edition.

134 *"For the person whose pain"*: Scarry, *Body in Pain*, 4.

134 *"About four o'clock, the army"*: Maupassant, "The First Snowfall," 252.

135 *"The animal was depressed"*: London, "To Build a Fire," 284.

136 *called an "interpretant"*: Peirce, *Collected Papers*, vol. 2, 136–37, 274.

137 *"I have given a name"*: Nietzsche, *Gay Science*, 249.

138 *being is never directed*: For more on Merleau-Ponty's particular brand of phenomenology, see Hammond, Howarth, and Keat, *Understanding Phenomenology*; Madison, *Phenomenology of Merleau-Ponty*; and M. Langer, *Merleau-Ponty's Phenomenology of Perception*.

140 *"The object 'speaks'"*: Merleau-Ponty, *Phenomenology of Perception*, 131.

140 *"To get used to a hat"*: Ibid., 132.

141 *"My doppelganger"*: Daudet, *In the Land of Pain*, 61.

142 *"The road could hardly be seen"*: Tolstoy, "Master and Man," 459–60, 467, 487, 491. All subsequent quotations from this story are taken from this edition.

144 *"The object is treated as a subject"*: Culler, *Pursuit of Signs*, 142.

145 *"It may seem strange"*: S. Langer, *Mind*, 24.

145 *"the movement of emotive"*: Ibid., 29.

146 *"like the socket of a pulled tooth"*: Doty, *Heaven's Coast*, 7.

146 *"helplessness and desolation"*: Ibid., 26–27.

147 *"When I saw Mister"*: Morrison, *Beloved*, 85–86.

148 *"Is there anybody like me"*: Garrison, *Don't Leave Me This Way*, 55.

148 *"I see him in my mind's eye"*: Daudet, *In the Land of Pain*, 56.

148 *"I was almost 42 years old"*: Hsi, *Closing the Chart*, 127.

149 *"The ship is sinking"*: Daudet, *In the Land of Pain*, 7.

149 *"No remembering now"*: Wiman, "After the Diagnosis."

150 *"Time . . . started to shudder"*: Garrison, *Don't Leave Me This Way*, 6.

151 *"At the beginning of the nineteenth"*: Foucault, *Birth of the Clinic*, xii.

152 *"By saying what one sees"*: Ibid., 114. Foucault also emphasizes the costs of our "oculocentric discourse." We may advance our collective understanding of disease by studying patients in the clinic, but we do so at the expense of those patients: "But to look in order to know, to show in order to teach, is not this a tacit form of violence, all the more abusive for its silence, upon a sick body that demands to be comforted, not displayed? Can pain be a spectacle?" (84).

152 *We pass by them*: Sartre, *Being and Nothingness*, 328, 330.

152 *"that the Other accomplishes for us"*: Ibid., 353–54. See also Lacan, *Ecrits*, 2, 86, 141. While Sartre, Foucault, and Lacan point to the positive side of acquiring knowledge through the other, they also want to emphasize its negative one—in particular its profoundly alienating nature. For example, the body that we come to know by adopting the other's point of view is *not our own*.

153 *Certain neurons in the brains of monkeys*: For more on the science of mirror neurons and its implications, see Iacoboni, *Mirroring People*, and Rizzolati and Sinigaglia, *Mirrors in the Brain*.

154 *our greatest collective achievements*: Proof that mirror neurons foster social skills and behavior also comes from diseases like autism, in which a dysfunctional mirroring system may be responsible for severe social deficits. See Iacoboni, *Mirroring People*, 157–83.

154 *Dalai Lama neurons*: Ramachandran, "The Neurology of Self-Awareness," 3.

155 *"I had suddenly stopped"*: Karinthy, *Journey Round My Skull*, 59.

156 *"If worlds are made"*: Goodman, *Ways of Worldmaking*, 22.

158 *central to all creative acts*: See Scarry, *Body in Pain*, 281–307.

159 *"The general distribution of material objects"*: Ibid., 291.

159 *"The simple triad"*: Ibid., 39.

160 *Crane's survivors enlarge, color*: There are many ways to make—or, more accurately, to remake—our worlds, as Goodman suggests, including composition and decomposition, weighting, ordering, supplementation and deletion, and deformation (*Ways of Worldmaking*, 7–17).

160 *Consider the house*: Morrison, *Beloved*, 10–11, 35.

161 *"cloth-covered sheepskin coat"*: Tolstoy, "Master and Man," 457. All subsequent quotations from this story are taken from this edition.

163 *"rooted deep"*: Crane, "The Open Boat," 69. All subsequent quotations from this story are taken from this edition.

164 *"If one imagines"*: Scarry, *Body in Pain*, 289–90.

Chapter 9: The X-Ray

167 *the "night-side" of life*: Sontag, *Illness as Metaphor*, 3.

168 *"It was coughing"*: Mann, *Magic Mountain*, 12, 13.

168 *"extravagant thrill of joy"*: Ibid., 89, 92.

168   *"swimming jellyfish"*: Ibid., 217.

168   *"And Hans Castorp saw"*: Ibid., 218–19.

169   *the making visible*: Foucault, *Birth of the Clinic*, xii, 51, 64, 114–15.

171   *Our relative detachment*: In order to maximize survival, the body is designed
       to prioritize engagement with the outside world and minimize engagement
       with the inside one. We saw that in our discussions of perception as pri-
       marily perception of the outside world. But the nervous system as a whole
       similarly can be said to "face outward." Consider the following neuroana-
       tomical facts: (1) the nervous system arises from the same area in the
       embryo as the skin, the ectoderm, which is located at the boundary
       between the inside and outside worlds; (2) the majority of the mature brain
       is involved in the sensory and motor capacities of speech and perception;
       (3) within these critical areas, our self-image (homunculus) is formed—a
       dynamic image that depends on ongoing stimuli from our external environ-
       ments; and (4) the self-image represents areas of the body disproportion-
       ately, our hands and feet (body parts engaged in surveying the environment)
       taking up over half the image. At the same time, the hypothalamus—the
       part of the brain that controls (automatically and silently) the activity of
       our vital internal organs—makes up less than 1 percent of the brain.
       According to Irving Kupferman, even consciousness, a phenomenon so
       apparently representative of our *inner* lives, may have evolved primarily to
       deal with the external world (so much more unpredictable than the inter-
       nal one) more effectively. See Kandel and Schwartz, *Principles of Neural
       Science*, 322–23, 612, 624.

172   *"so vague and muddy"*: Miller, *Body in Question*, 42.

173   *Frida Kahlo may be the best example*: For insight into the connection
       between Kahlo's pain and her creativity, see Herrera's excellent biogra-
       phy, *Frida*, as well as the artist's own *Diary of Frida Kahlo*.

176   *"My painting"*: Herrera, *Frida*, 148.

176   *guided imagery and visualization*: See Simonton et al., *Getting Well
       Again*, and Lewandoski et al., "Changes in the Meaning of Pain."

178   *"red hot swords"*: Cited in Padfield, *Perceptions of Pain*, 60.

178   *"When I first saw"*: Ibid., 33.

180   *"When I wake up"*: Ibid., 118.

181   *"And his breath began to fail"*: Tolstoy, "How Much Land Does a Man
       Need?" 435.

182   *"Draw breath, Jo"*: Dickens, *Bleak House*, 692.

182 *"To Mr. Jarndyce"*: Ibid., 699–700.

182 *"For the cart"*: Ibid., 703.

183 *"I'm a-moving"*: Ibid., 690.

183 *"no heed of the course"*: London, "Love of Life," 173. All subsequent quotations from this story are taken from this edition.

184 *"The subjective experience"*: Miller, *The Body in Question*, 9–10.

184 *simple substitution metaphors*: For a discussion on the differences between substitution and interaction, as well as other theories on how metaphor works, see Black, *Models and Metaphors*, 219–37; Ricoeur, *Rule of Metaphor*, 44–133; and Soskice, *Metaphor and Religious Language*, 24–51.

185 *"The unmentionable odour"*: Auden, "September 1, 1939," in *Selected Poems*, 86.

187 *speculative instruments*: Richards, *Speculative Instruments*, 33–34, 46–48.

187 *is it a metaphorical seeing*: While most theorists believe that metaphor moves beyond language—after all, it is so often unparaphrasable—they are wary of attributing this capacity to mental imagery. Instead, Langer argues that metaphor engages in "presentational symbolism" and "abstractive seeing," which it shares with music and other nondiscursive art forms (*Philosophy in a New Key*, 98, 218, 141, 233); and Ricoeur speaks of a logical/verbal moment and a sensible/nonverbal one, which cooperate in metaphor's "work of resemblance" (*Rule of Metaphor*, 173–215).

187 *"The application of a label"*: Goodman, *Languages of Art*, 32.

187 *"the artist must make use"*: Ibid., 33.

188 *"Your body's center"*: Garrison, *Don't Leave Me This Way*, 45.

189 *"In fact, the entire"*: Ibid., 45.

189 *"My brain, which allowed me"*: Ibid., 47.

190 *"unprotected high cheekbones"*: London, "To Build a Fire," 283. All subsequent quotations from this story are taken from this edition.

192 *network of wires*: London was not the first person to use this metaphor. As Laura Otis discusses in her book *Networking* (23–25), the prominent French neuroscientist Emil Dubos-Raymond spoke of the nervous system in terms of the telegraph—a metaphorical model that he relied on to construct his theories about nerve-impulse transmission.

193 *"Our body is not in space"*: Merleau-Ponty, *Primacy of Perception*, 5.

195   *"But what is pain?"*: Heidegger, *Poetry, Language, Thought*, 204.

195   *The positive side of pain*: See Melzack and Wall, *Challenge of Pain*, 23–24.

196   *"move heaven and earth"*: Cousins, *Anatomy of an Illness*, 107.

197   *"Physicians too readily claim"*: Leriche, *Surgery of Pain*, 23.

199   *"living and life-producing"*: Cited in Abrams, *Mirror and the Lamp*, 172.

199   *"objective correlatives"*: Eliot, "Hamlet," 145.

199   *"muddy undersides and vulnerabilities"*: Hermann, *Cure for Grief*, 11.

199   *"To-day she could almost feel"*: Lawrence, *Lady Chatterley's Lover*, 113–14, 129.

201   *"[Pavel Ivanych] sleeps sitting"*: Chekhov, "Gusev," 254. All subsequent quotations from this story are taken from this edition.

202   *"'Last night,' said Sloppy"*: Dickens, *Our Mutual Friend*, 379.

203   *"'Did he just drop down'"*: Brand, "Wine on the Desert," 27. All subsequent quotations from this story are taken from this edition.

208   *"[The] very fact that a person"*: Scarry, *Body in Pain*, 255–56.

210   *"does not begin to exist"*: Merleau-Ponty, *Phenomenology of Perception*, 27–28.

210   *"A thought limited"*: Ibid., 177.

211   *"There is no 'private order'"*: Blackburn, "How to Refer to Private Experience," 201.

211   *"Language leads us to a thought"*: Merleau-Ponty, *Primacy of Perception*, 8.

Postscript

217   *"Litvak stood up slowly"*: Chabon, *The Yiddish Policemen's Union*, 347.

218   *"Their ceaseless talk"*: Scarry, *Body in Pain*, 33.

219   *As long as the conversation lasts*: Rorty, *Philosophy and the Mirror of Nature*, 318.

References

Abrams, M. H. *The Mirror and the Lamp: Romantic Theory and the Critical Tradition*. New York: Oxford University Press, 1953.

American Pain Society. *Pain: Current Understanding of Assessment, Management, and Treatments*. 2001. www.ampainsoc.org.

Arendt, Hannah. *The Human Condition*. Chicago: University of Chicago Press, 1998.

Aristotle. *Poetics*. In *The Complete Works of Aristotle: The Revised Oxford Translation*. Edited by J. Barnes. Princeton, NJ: Princeton University Press, 1984.

Armstrong, D. M. *Bodily Sensations*. London: Routledge, 1962.

———. *A Materialist Theory of Mind*. New York: Humanities, 1968.

Auden, W. H. *Selected Poems*. Edited by Edward Mendelson. New York: Vintage International, 1989.

Bakan, David. *Disease, Pain, and Sacrifice: Towards a Psychology of Suffering*. Chicago: University of Chicago Press, 1968.

Bauby, Jean-Dominique. *The Diving Bell and the Butterfly*. New York: Vintage, 1998.

Beecher, Henry K. "Pain in Men Wounded in Battle." *Annals of Surgery* 123, no.1 (1946).

Black, Max. *Models and Metaphors*. Ithaca: Cornell University Press, 1962.

———. "More about Metaphor." In *Metaphor and Thought*. Edited by Andrew Ortony. Cambridge: Cambridge University Press, 1979.

Blackburn, Simon. "How to Refer to Private Experience." In *Proceedings of the Aristotelian Society* 75 (1974–1975).

———. *Spreading the Word: Groundings in the Philosophy of Language*. Oxford: Oxford University Press, 1987.

Bolton, Derek. *An Approach to Wittgenstein's Philosophy*. London: Macmillan, 1979.

Boyd, Richard. "Metaphor and Theory Change." In *Metaphor and Thought*. Edited by Andrew Ortony. Cambridge: Cambridge University Press, 1979.

Brand, Max. "Wine on the Desert." In *Max Brand's Best Western Stories*. Edited by William Nolan. London: Robert Hale, 1981.

Burney, Fanny. *A Known Scribbler: Francis Burney on Literary Life*. Edited by Justine Crump. Peterborough, ON: Broadview Press, 2002.

Cassell, Eric. *The Nature of Suffering*. New York: Oxford University Press, 1991.

Cassirer, Ernst. *Language and Myth*. Translated by Susanne Langer. New York: Dover, 1953.

Chabon, Michael. *The Yiddish Policemen's Union*. New York: HarperCollins, 2007.

Chekhov, Anton. "Gusev." In *The Portable Chekhov*. Edited by Avraham Yarmolinsky. New York: Penguin, 1977.

———. "Heartache." In *The Portable Chekhov*.

Chisholm, Roderick. *Perceiving: A Philosophical Study*. Ithaca, NY: Cornell University Press, 1957.

———. "Sentences about Believing" in *Proceedings of the Aristotelian Society* 56 (1956).

Cleeland, Charles, et al. "Pain and Its Treatment in Patients with Metastatic Cancer," *New England Journal of Medicine* 330, no. 9 (1994).

Cousins, Norman. *Anatomy of an Illness*. New York: Bantam, 1981.

Crane, Stephen. "The Open Boat: A Tale intended to be after the Fact. Being the Experience of four men from the Sunk Steamer Commodore." In *The Works of Stephen Crane*. Edited by Fredson Bowers. Charlottesville: University Press of Virginia, 1970.

Culler, Jonathan. *The Pursuit of Signs*. Ithaca, NY: Cornell University Press, 1981.

Daudet, Alphonse. *In the Land of Pain*. Edited and translated by Julian Barnes. New York: Knopf, 2002.

Davidson, Donald. "What Metaphors Mean." In *On Metaphor*. Edited by Sheldon Sacks. Chicago: University of Chicago Press, 1979.

de Man, Paul. *Allegories of Reading*. New Haven, CT: Yale University Press, 1979.

Derrida, Jacques. "White Mythology." Translated by F. C. T. Moore. In *New Literary History* 6, no. 1 (1974).

Dickens, Charles. *Bleak House*. Edited by Norman Page. Harmondsworth, UK: Penguin, 1971.

———. *Hard Times*. London: Geoffrey Cumberlege, 1955.

———. *Our Mutual Friend*. Edited by J. Hillis Miller. Harmondsworth, UK: Penguin, 1971.

Dickinson, Emily. *The Complete Poems of Emily Dickinson*. Edited by T. H. Johnson. Boston: Little, Brown, 1955.

Didion, Joan, *The White Album*. New York: Farrar, Straus and Giroux, 1990.

———. *The Year of Magical Thinking*. New York: Knopf, 2005.

Donne, John. *Devotions upon Emergent Occasions and Death's Duel*. Preface by Andrew Motion. New York: Vintage, 1999.

Doty, Mark. *Heaven's Coast*. New York: HarperPerennial, 1997.

Edson, Margaret. *Wit*. New York: Faber and Faber, 1999.

Eliot, T. S. "Hamlet." In *Collected Essays*. London: Faber and Faber, 1932.

Faulkner, William. Nobel Prize acceptance speech, 1950. www.nobelprize.org.

Foucault, Michel. *The Birth of the Clinic*. Translated by A. M. Sheridan Smith. New York: Vintage, 1973.

Frankl, Viktor. *Man's Search for Meaning*. New York: Pocket, 1985.

Freud, Sigmund. "Inhibitions, Symptoms, and Anxiety." In *The Standard Edition of the Complete Philosophical Works of Sigmund Freud*. Edited and translated by James Strachey, Anna Freud, A. Strachey, and A. Tyson. London: Hogarth, 1959.

———. "Mourning and Melancholia." In *The Standard Edition of the Complete Philosophical Works of Sigmund Freud*.

Frye, Northrop. *Anatomy of Criticism*. Princeton, NJ: Princeton University Press, 1957.

Garrison, Julia Fox. *Don't Leave Me This Way: Or When I Get Back on My Feet You'll Be Sorry*. New York: HarperCollins, 2007.

Goodman, Nelson. *Languages of Art*. Indianapolis: Hackett, 1976.

———. *Ways of Worldmaking*. Indianapolis: Hackett, 1978.

Grahek, Nikola. *Feeling Pain and Being in Pain*. Cambridge: MIT Press, 2007.

Grealy, Lucy. *Autobiography of a Face*. New York: HarperPerennial, 2003.

Greenberg, Michael. *Hurry Down Sunshine*. New York: Other Press, 2008.

Hacker, P. M. S. *Insight and Illusion*. Oxford: Clarendon, 1986.

Hacker, P. M. S., and G. Baker. *Scepticism, Rules and Meaning*. Oxford: Blackwell, 1984.

Hammond, M., J. Howarth, and R. Keat. *Understanding Phenomenology*. Oxford: Blackwell, 1991.

Hampton, Tracy. "A World of Pain: Scientists Explore Factors Controlling Pain Perception." *Journal of the American Medical Association* 296, no. 20 (2006).

Hardy, Thomas. *The Woodlanders*. Edited by Dale Kramer. Oxford: Clarendon, 1981.

Heidegger, Martin. *Poetry, Language, Thought*. Translated by Albert Hofstadter. New York: Harper & Row, 1971.

Hemingway, Ernest. "The Snows of Kilimanjaro." In *The Essential Hemingway*. Harmondsworth, UK: Penguin, 1947.

Henle, Paul. "Language, Thought, and Culture." In *Language, Thought, and Culture*. Edited by Paul Henle. Ann Arbor: University of Michigan Press, 1958.

Hermann, Nellie. *The Cure for Grief*. New York: Scribner, 2008.

Herrera, Hayden. *Frida: A Biography of Frida Kahlo*. New York: HarperPerennial, 2002.

Hesse, Mary. *Models and Analogies in Science*. Notre Dame, IN: University of Notre Dame Press, 1970.

Hester, Marcus. *The Meaning of Poetic Metaphor*. The Hague: Mouton, 1967.

Hsi, Steven D. *Closing the Chart: A Dying Physician Examines Family, Faith, and Medicine*. Albuquerque: University of New Mexico Press, 2004.

Iacoboni. Marco. *Mirroring People: The New Science of How We Connect with Others*. New York: Farrar, Straus and Giroux, 2008.

International Association for the Study of Pain Subcommittee on Taxonomy. "Pain Terms: A List with Definitions and Notes on Usage." *Pain* 6, no. 3 (1979).

James, William. *The Work of William James: The Principles of Psychology.* Edited by F. H. Burkhardt et al. Cambridge, MA: Harvard University Press, 1981.

Jamison, Kay Redfield. *An Unquiet Mind: A Memoir of Moods and Madness.* New York: Vintage, 1995.

Johnson, Mark. *The Body in the Mind.* Chicago: University of Chicago Press, 1987.

Johnson, Mark, and George Lakoff. *Metaphors We Live By.* Chicago: University of Chicago Press, 1980.

Joyce, James. *A Portrait of the Artist as a Young Man.* In *The Portable James Joyce.* Edited by Harry Levin. New York: Penguin, 1946.

Kahlo, Frida. *The Diary of Frida Kahlo: An Intimate Self-Portrait.* Translated by Barbara Toledo and Ricardo Pohlenz. New York: Abrams, 1995.

Kandel, Eric, and James Schwartz. *Principles of Neural Science.* New York: Elsevier, 1985.

Karinthy, Frigyes. *A Journey Round My Skull.* Translated by Vernon Barker. Budapest: Corvina, 1992.

Kripke, S. A. *Wittgenstein on Rules and Private Language.* Oxford: Blackwell, 1986.

Lacan, Jacques. *Ecrits: A Selection.* Translated by Alan Sheridan Smith. New York: Norton, 1977.

Langer, Monika. *Merleau-Ponty's Phenomenology of Perception: A Guide and Commentary.* London: Macmillan, 1989.

Langer, Susanne. *Mind: An Essay on Human Feeling.* Abridged edition. Edited by G. V. D. Heuval. Baltimore: Johns Hopkins University Press, 1989.

———. *Philosophy in a New Key.* Cambridge, MA: Harvard University Press, 1957.

Larue, F., et al. "Underestimation and Undertreatment of Pain in HIV Disease." *British Medical Journal* 314 (1997).

Lawrence, D. H. *Lady Chatterley's Lover.* New York: NALPenguin, 1959.

Leriche, René. *The Surgery of Pain.* Baltimore: Williams and Wilkins, 1939.

Levertov, Denise. *The Freeing of the Dust.* New York: New Directions, 1972.

Lewandowski, Wendy, et al. "Changes in the Meaning of Pain with the Uses of Guided Imagery." *Pain Management Nursing* 6, no. 2 (2005).

London, Jack. "To Build a Fire." In *Short Stories of Jack London.* Edited by Earle Labor, Robert Leitz, and I. M. Shepard. New York: Collier, 1991.

———. "The Heathen." In *Short Stories of Jack London.*

———. "The House of Mapui." In *Short Stories of Jack London.*

———. "Love of Life." In *Short Stories of Jack London.*

———. "The White Silence." In *Short Stories of Jack London.*

Mac Cormac, Earl. *A Cognitive Theory of Metaphor*. Cambridge: MIT Press, 1985.

Madison, Gary Brent. *The Phenomenology of Merleau-Ponty*. Athens: Ohio University Press, 1981.

Maimonides, Moses. *The Guide for the Perplexed*. Translated by Shlomo Pines. Chicago: University of Chicago Press, 1963.

Malcolm, Norman. *Nothing Is Hidden*. Oxford: Blackwell, 1986.

Mann, Thomas, *The Magic Mountain*. Translated by H. T. Lowe-Porter. New York: Random House, 1952.

Marks, Richard, and Edward J. Sacher. "Undertreatment of Medical Inpatients with Narcotic Analgesics." *Annals of Internal Medicine* 78, no. 2 (1973).

Maupassant, Guy de. "The First Snowfall." In *Short Stories of the Comedy and Tragedy of Life by Guy de Maupassant*. London: M. Walker Dunne, 1903.

Mayor, Susan. "Survey of Patients Shows That Cancer Pain Still Undertreated." *British Medical Journal* 321 (2000).

McGinn, C. *Wittgenstein on Meaning*. Oxford: Blackwell, 1984.

Medvei, V. C. *The Mental and Physical Effects of Pain*. Edinburgh: Livingstone, 1949.

Melzack, Ronald. "The McGill Pain Questionnaire." *Pain* 1 (1975).

———. *The Puzzle of Pain*. New York: Basic Books, 1973.

Melzack, Ronald, and Patrick Wall. *The Challenge of Pain*. New York: Basic Book, 1983.

Merleau-Ponty, Maurice. *The Phenomenology of Perception*. Translated by Colin Smith. London: Routledge & Kegan Paul, 1962.

———. *The Primacy of Perception and Other Essays on Phenomenological Psychology, the Philosophy of Art, History, and Politics*. Edited by James Edie. Evanston, IL: Northwestern University Press, 1964.

Miller, Jonathan. *The Body in Question*. New York: Vintage, 1982.

Mitchell, Joyce Slayton. *Winning the Chemo Battle*. New York: Norton, 1988.

Moore, Lorrie. "To Fill." In *Self-Help: Stories*. New York: Vintage, 2007.

Morgan, John. "America Opiophobia: Customary Underutilization of Opioid Analgesics." In *Advances in Pain Research and Therapy*. Edited by C. S. Hill and William Fields. New York: Raven, 1989.

Morris, David. *The Culture of Pain*. Berkeley: University of California Press, 1991.

———. *Illness and Culture*. Berkeley: University of California Press, 2000.

Morrison, Toni. *Beloved*. New York: Vintage, 2004.

Nietzsche, Friedrich. *The Gay Science*. Translated by Walter Kaufmann. New York: Vintage, 1974.

———. *The Will to Power*. In *The Complete Works of Friedrich Nietzsche*. Edited by Oscar Levy. Translated by Anthony Ludovici. New York: Russell and Russell, 1910.

Ortony, Andrew, ed. *Metaphor and Thought*. Cambridge: Cambridge University Press, 1979.

Otis, Laura. *Networking: Communicating with Bodies and Machines in the Nineteenth Century*. Ann Arbor: University of Michigan Press, 2001.

Padfield, Deborah. *Perceptions of Pain*. Stockport, UK: Dewi Lewis, 2003.

Pears, David. *The False Prison: A Study of the Development of Wittgenstein's Philosophy*. Oxford: Oxford University Press, 1988.

Peirce, C. S. *Collected Papers*. Edited by C. Hartshorne, P. Weiss, and A. W. Burks. Cambridge, MA: Harvard University Press, 1931–1958.

Pinker, Steven. *The Stuff of Thought: Language as a Window into Human Nature*. New York: Penguin, 2008.

Pitcher, George. *The Philosophy of Wittgenstein*. Englewood Cliffs, NJ: Prentice-Hall, 1964.

Price, Reynolds. *A Whole New Life: An Illness and a Healing*. New York: Scribner, 1982.

Proulx, Annie. "The Mud Below." In *Close Range: Wyoming Stories*. New York: Scribner, 2003.

Quine, W. V. "A Postscript on Metaphor." In *On Metaphor*. Edited by Sheldon Sacks. Chicago: University of Chicago Press, 1978.

Quintilian. *Institutio Oratoria*. Translated by H. E. Butler. London: Heinemann, 1920.

Radner, Gilda. *It's Always Something*. New York: Avon, 1989.

Ramachandran, V. S. "The Neurology of Self-Awareness." January 2007. www.edge.org.

Richards, I. A. *Speculative Instruments*. London: Routledge & Kegan Paul, 1955.

Ricoeur, Paul. *The Rule of Metaphor*. Translated by Robert Czerny. Toronto: University of Toronto Press, 1975.

Rizzolatti, Giacomo, and Corrado Sinigaglia. *Mirrors in the Brain: How Our Minds Share Actions, Emotions, and Experience*. New York: Oxford University Press, 2008.

Rorty, Richard. *Contingency, Irony, and Solidarity*. New York: Cambridge University Press, 1989.

———. *Philosophy and the Mirror of Nature*. Princeton, NJ: Princeton University Press, 1979.

Ryan, Cornelius, and Kathryn Morgan Ryan. *A Private Battle*. New York: Fawcett, 1979.

Ryle, Gilbert. *The Concept of Mind*. London: Hutchinson's Library, 1949.

Sacks, Oliver. *A Leg to Stand On*. New York: Touchstone, 1998.

Sartre, Jean-Paul. *Being and Nothingness*. Translated by Hazel Barnes. New York: Philosophical Library, 1956.

Scarry, Elaine. *The Body in Pain*. New York: Oxford University Press, 1985.

————. "Introduction." In *Literature and the Body: Essays on Populations and Persons*, Edited by Elaine Scarry. Baltimore: Johns Hopkins University Press, 1988.

Searle, John. *Intentionality*. Cambridge: Cambridge University Press, 1983.

Shaw, Bernard, *The Doctor's Dilemma*. Harmondsworth, UK: Penguin, 1946.

Shkolvsky, Victor. "Art as Technique." In *Modern Criticism and Theory*. Edited by David Lodge. Translated by L. T. Lemon and M. Reis. London: Longman, 1988.

Simonton, O. Carl, Stephanie Matthews-Simonton, and James Creighton. *Getting Well Again*. New York: Vintage, 1977.

Solzhenitsyn, Alexander. *Cancer Ward*. Translated by Nicholas Bethell and David Berg. New York: Bantam, 1969.

Sontag, Susan. *Illness as Metaphor*. New York: Vintage, 1977.

Sophocles. *Philoctetes*. In *The Complete Greek Tragedies: Sophocles II*. Edited by David Green and Richard Lattimore. Translated by David Green. Chicago: University of Chicago Press, 1957.

Soskice, Janice Martin. *Metaphor and Religious Language*. Oxford: Clarendon, 1985.

Stephens, James. "The Wind." In *The Norton Anthology of Modern Poetry*. Edited by Richard Ellmann and Robert O'Clair. New York: Norton, 1973.

Sternbach, Richard. *Pain: A Psychophysiological Analysis*. New York: Academic Press, 1968.

Styron, William. *Darkness Visible: A Memoir of Madness*. New York: Vintage, 1992.

Tolstoy, Leo. "How Much Land Does a Man Need?" In *Tolstoy's Tales of Courage and Conflict*. Edited by Charles Neider. Translated by Nathan Dole. New York: Hanover House, 1958.

————. "Lost on the Steppe." In *Tolstoy's Tales of Courage and Conflict*.

————. "Master and Man." In *Great Short Works of Leo Tolstoy*. Translated by Louise and Alymer Maude. New York: Perennial Library, 1967.

Trigg, Roger. *Pain and Emotion*. Oxford: Clarendon, 1970.

Tye, Michael. *Ten Problems of Consciousness: A Representational Theory of the Phenomenal Mind*. Cambridge, MA: MIT Press, 1995.

U. S. Department of Health and Human Services. *Management of Cancer Pain*. Washington, DC: U.S. Department of Health and Human Services, 1994.

Wallace, David Foster. "The Depressed Person." *Harper's Magazine*, January 1998.

Walzer, Michael. *Just and Unjust Wars: A Moral Argument with Historical Illustrations*. New York: Basic, 1977.

Wiman, Christian. "After the Diagnosis." *The New Yorker*, March 12, 2007.

Wittgenstein, Ludwig. *The Blue and Brown Books*. New York: Harper and Row, 1958.

————. *Philosophical Investigations*. Edited by G. E. M. Anscombe, R. Rhees, and G. H. von Wright. Translated by G. E. M. Anscombe. Oxford: Blackwell, 1958.

————. *Remarks on the Philosophy of Psychology*. Edited by G. E. M. Anscombe and G. H. von Wright. Translated by G. E. M Anscombe. Oxford: Blackwell, 1980.

————. *Tractatus Logico-Philosophicus*. Translated by D. F. Pears and B. McGuinness. London: Routledge & Kegan Paul, 1961.

————. *Wittgenstein's Lectures, Cambridge, 1932–35*. Edited by Alice Ambrose. Oxford: Blackwell, 1979.

————. *Zettel*. Edited by G. E. M. Anscombe and G. H. von Wright. Translated by G. E. M. Anscombe. Oxford: Blackwell, 1967.

Woolf, Virginia. "On Being Ill." In *Collected Essays*. New York: Harcourt, 1967.

Acknowledgments

This book had a long gestation period and there are many people who helped me along the way I wish to thank.

The first phase began in medical school after reading *The Body in Pain*. Elaine Scarry's book deeply moved me and made me want to respond, even replicate—for a thing of beauty, Scarry says, always prompts the desire to replicate. I decided to start with the same premise—that pain is inexpressible—and instead of panning outward like Scarry, I would follow its implications on a smaller, more intimate scale. What does the running dry of language mean for the person in pain and how can we restore its flow? I was encouraged by David Rothman and Stephanie Kiceluk at the Institute for the Study of Society and Medicine at Columbia to pursue these questions. Along with my parents and close friend Susie Holloway, they convinced me that there was room in medicine for doctors who were passionate about language and literature.

The next phase took place at Oxford, where I had the incredible fortune to have Terry Eagleton as my dissertation adviser. Although he is best known for his books on literary theory, Terry's greatest skill may well be in the less celebrated realm of teaching. After a devastating (though accurate) assault on some preliminary chapters, Terry explained precisely what was needed to elevate my work to the graduate level. For the next few years, despite his ludicrously busy schedule, Terry was always available, always enthusiastic, and always insightful. I will forever treasure the time I spent with him. As I will the time I spent with my three best friends at Oxford and fellow members of the Galen Society: Jillian Kearney, Shannon Russell, and Rohinie Jayatilaka.

The final phase began after the project emerged from a prolonged slumber. I had been busy finishing medical training, loving my beautiful wife Daniella, and enjoying life in New York City. But Scarry and her ideas continued to buzz in my head and would grow louder during an unexpected bout with serious illness at the end of my residency. So a decade after receiving my doctorate, I retrieved my thesis from the back of the bookshelf. Not the elegant, important work I remembered, it was in fact a monster, insufferably long and virtually unreadable. It would need a major overhaul if I ever wanted anyone besides graduate students to make sense of it. Mert Erogul and Kathy Powderly encouraged me at the time to make the language of pain a part of the medicine and literature elective we taught together at Downstate Medical School. I began paring down and revising the monster. Eric Hoffmann, a close friend and gifted educator at CUNY, graciously read through the book and made key suggestions. As did Sandy Gruenwald, who acted as a de facto agent, making calls to everyone she knew in every part of the world. David Rothenberg and Steven Fisch, who slyly floated the idea of a possible movie (I have funny friends), were equally supportive at this early stage. As was Judith Rabkin, a psychiatry professor at Columbia who shares my love for Fire Island sunsets, and David Elpern, the William Osler of dermatology who has been a mentor to me in the medical humanities. I also want to thank Professors Rita Charon, Sayantani Dasgupta, Nellie Hermann, and Austin Zubin for their helpful comments and encouragement.

By far my biggest stroke of luck came when Quang Bao was appointed director of the Rema Hort Mann Foundation, where I had been managing the cancer wing. We became instant friends because of our mutual passion for literature and theater. After reading my book, Q became its most ardent supporter. Unfazed by the fact that no agent wanted anything to do with me, Q remained determined. The man was tireless, especially when my spirits flagged, and eventually, through his efforts, I found Kirby Kim, another believer and rare bird in the literary business—as interested in words and ideas as he is in money and success. KK, thank you so much for helping me make my monster look halfway presentable. I am so grateful to have you and Q as friends.

Above all, I want to thank Amy Cherry at Norton. When I got back her first round of edits, I confess I was alarmed—there was more red ink on the pages than my words. But I quickly realized how valuable her exacting criticism would be. Even more important, Amy helped me transform what was originally a theoretical work into a much more concrete and practical one—which of course it had to be since pain isn't an abstract part of our lives but an all too real part. I am thrilled with how the final version turned out—Is it really the final version? Can it be after all these years?—thanks in large measure to Amy's insights, attention to detail, and generosity with her time and energy.

For the finishing touches, I want to thank Liz Duvall for tracking down and correcting all my mistakes; Ellen Tien, a magician with words, who helped (as she always does) invigorate my prose; Erica Stern, who steered me, with patience and humor, through the entire publication process; and Donna Maddalena, Grace LaSelva, and Julianne DiBenedetto, who helped me with the permissions and images.

Finally, I am grateful for the ongoing personal support. Thank you to my friends, who year after year never failed to inquire about "the book" that never quite seemed to materialize. Mercifully I no longer have to lower my eyes and change the subject. All done, I can now say—FINALLY! Thank you also to my parents and sisters and brothers-in-law for their selfless love. And of course to Daniella and our two magnificent boys, Luca and Daniel—my three greatest sources of inspiration.

Text Credits

Index

Page numbers in *italics* refer to illustrations.

"After the Diagnosis" (Wiman), 149–50
agency, language of, 16, 41–42, 70–71,
    72, 76–77, 79–96, 97, 114–15,
    125–28, 173, 174, 207, 215,
    216
  aversiveness captured by, 92–93
  injury and, 89–90, 94–96
  in McGill Pain Questionnaire, 13,
    80–82, *81*, 83, 158
  military metaphor in, 84–88, 92, 94,
    123, 124
  narrative of, 91–92, *91*, 94, *94*
  problems of, 124
  signaling aspect of, 103–7, 110, 135
  types of, 116
agency, literary, 97–128
  cold as, 98, 101–3, 106, 107, 116–17,
    134–36, 139, 142–44
  force in, 110–17, 127
  foreshadowing in, 103–6, 112
  intention in, 118–28
  ocean waves as, 108–10, 115, 120–
    21, 127, 163
  personification in, 118–24, 128
  physicality in, 111–16, 128
  readers as observers of, 100, 101, 103,
    107, 109–10, 113, 135–36
  threat in, 99–110, 127, 128, 135–37,
    227*n*
  voice acquired by, 107–9, 110, 118,
    128, 142, 163
  wind as, 107, 108, 112–15, 117, 120–
    21, 127
AIDS, 85, 98, 133, 146, 222*n*
altitude sickness, 170–71

American Pain Society, 221*n*
anatomic metaphors, 16, 167–211, 215,
    217
  in art, 173–76, *175*, 197–99, *198*
  in art therapy, 176–80, *177, 178, 179*
  imaging the body in, 170–80
  projection metaphors as, 197–206
Anatomy of an Illness (Cousins), 196
angina, 82, 114–15
ankylosing spondylitis, 196
appendicitis, 79, 80, 85
Arendt, Hannah, 23
Aristotle, 71, 73, 185
artifacts, 157–66, 197, 207
  as substitution metaphors, 181–87
art therapy, 176–80, *177, 178, 179*
Auden, W. H., 14, 28, 32, 83, 98, 185
Autobiography of a Face (Grealy), 104
Aversiveness of pain, 92–93, 98, 122,
    162, 217

Bakan, David, 46–47
battlefield injuries, 42
Bauby, Jean-Dominique, 25, 26, 60, 61,
    138
Beecher, Henry, 42
being-in-the-world, concept of, 25,
    26–27, 41, 54, 153, 171, 221*n*
Beloved (Morrison), 96, 97, 146–47,
    160–61
bipolar disorder, 30–31
Birth of the Clinic, The (Foucault),
    151–52
Black, Max, 185, 188, 225*n*
Blackburn, Simon, 210–11

Bleak House (Dickens), 182–83
body, 132, 159–60, 161, 186
  homunculus of, 193, 231*n*
  pain caused by responses of, 116–17
  progressive fragmentation of, 138
  responses to altitude in, 170–71
  responses to cold in, 190–94
  sensory organs of, 45–46, 170
  sexual aspects of, 199–200
  tools as extensions of, 140, 158,
    163–64
  X-rays of, 168–69, 172
  see also anatomic metaphors
body, inaccessibility of, 16, 43–47, 53,
    54, 168–73, 200, 217
  automatic internal processes in,
    170–71
  inability to check with outside sources
    in, 45, 46, 69, 170
  individual intuitive awareness of body
    vs., 44, 45
  inherent indeterminacy of sensation
    in, 45–46, 69, 170
  perceptual limitations in, 45, 46, 69,
    170
  projection metaphors and, 150–53
Body in the Mind, The (Johnson), 111
brain, 157–58, 188–89, 191, 195, 231*n*
  mirror neurons in, 153–57
  perception of pain in, 42–43, 94–95
brain tumors, 154–55
Brand, Max (Frederick Faust), 202–6
Brand, Paul, 196
Broken Column, The (Kahlo), 175–76,
    175, 181, 185, 197
Bronze Age figurines, 199
Buddhism, 214

Burney, Fanny, 82–83, 92, 104, 116

Camus, Albert, 29, 31, 106
cancer, cancer patients, 34–35, 98, 104,
    117, 121–22, 133, 134, 172,
    197, 214
  art therapy for, 176–80, 177
  guided visualization technique for, 176

spinal cord, 83–84
  war and, 86–87, 92, 94, 128
Cancer Ward (Solzhenitsyn), 27, 87
cardiac patients, 82, 114–15, 124, 128
Cassell, Eric, 105–6
Cassirer, Ernst, 77
Castorp, Hans (char.), 167–69, 170–72
catachresis, 73–77, 186
Chabon, Michael, 217, 218
Chekhov, Anton, 60, 200–201, 202
chemotherapeutic agents, 86–87
Chisholm, Roderick, 223*n*
chronic pain syndromes, 14, 36–37,
    42, 58, 80, 96, 104, 124, 177,
    221*n*
Closing the Chart (Hsi), 84
Coleridge, Samuel, 199
communication, desire for, 20, 31,
    56–61, 90
Concept of Mind, The (Ryle), 65
Cousins, Norman, 196, 197
Crane, Stephen, 98, 108–10, 128, 160,
    163–64, 165, 166, 215
Culler, Jonathan, 144
Cure for Grief, The (Hermann), 167, 199

Dalai Lama, 154
Darkness Visible (Styron), 18–19, 29,
    37–38
Daudet, Alphonse, 18, 19, 20, 83, 92,
    104, 141, 148, 151, 156, 165,
    174, 215
Davidson, Donald, 71
Dedalus, Stephen (char.), 65–66, 68–70,
    72, 78, 88, 89, 136, 180
deformity, 104
del Duca, Simone, 37–38
de Man, Paul, 124, 125
depression, 14, 18–19, 29, 104, 115–16,
    214, 218, 223*n*
  descriptive elusiveness of, 37–38,
    40–41
  friends' insensitivity to, 31
  manic, 96
  pain as cause of, 37
Derrida, Jacques, 224*n*–25*n*

Descartes, René, 44, 54, 94, 139, 208
Devotions on Emergent Occasions
    (Donne), 85
diabetes, 103, 196
Dickens, Charles, 182–83, 188, 201–2
Dickinson, Emily, 14, 16, 17, 36, 37, 39,
    57–58, 59, 123
Didion, Joan, 18–19, 20, 58–59, 96, 106
Diving Bell and the Butterfly, The
    (Bauby), 25, 60
"Divorcing" (Levertov), 106
Doctor's Dilemma, The (Shaw), 85–86, 123
Donne, John, 59–60, 85
Don't Leave Me This Way (Garrison),
    147–48, 188–89
Doty, Mark, 146, 147, 151, 156
Dream, The (Kahlo), 174
Dubos-Raymond, Emil, 232*n*
Durante (char.), 202–6
dysesthesias, 83

Edson, Margaret, 123
Eliot, T. S., 199
Elusiveness of pain, descriptive, 15,
    36–47, 67–68, 119, 126, 136
  in depression, 37–38, 40–41
  inaccessibility of the body and, 43–47,
    54
  lack of intentionality and, 39–41, 47,
    54, 68
embodiment, 44, 207
  of consciousness, 110–11, 119, 139
epoché, concept of, 26–27, 29, 98, 106,
    130, 138, 142–43, 160, 215,
    218, 221*n*

Faces Pain Scale, 13–14, *13*, 80–82
Faulkner, William, 56, 57, 60
Faust, Frederick (Max Brand), 202–6
fellow sufferers, 115, 141, 145, 147–49,
    154, 165, 178–79, 213
Few Small Nips, A (Kahlo), 174
fibromyalgia, 42, 96, 104
"First Snowfall, The" (Maupassant),
    101–3, 107, 118, 134–35
Flaubert, Gustave, 156

force, in literary agency, 110–17, 127
foreshadowing, 103–6, 112
Foucault, Michel, 151–52, 169, 174,
    229*n*, 230*n*
Frankl, Viktor, 58, 61
Freud, Sigmund, 40–41, 104, 223*n*

Garrison, Julia Fox, 147–48, 150, 151,
    188–89, 192
Gary, Romain, 29, 31
genetic factors, 43, 95, 103, 121,
    155–56
George S (patient), 36–37, 38, 41, 56,
    58
germ theory, 85
Gillray, James, 121, *122*, 128
Gleevec, 87
God, 75, 123, 124
Goodman, Nelson, 19, 68, 132, 156,
    157, 185, 225*n*, 230*n*
gout, 121, *122*, 128
Grahek, Nikola, 227*n*
Grealy, Lucy, 104
Greenberg, Michael, 30–31
grief, 18–19, 41, 58–59, 60, 96, 104,
    106, 146, 167, 199, 214
guided imagery, 176
Guide for the Perplexed (Maimonides),
    75
"Gusev" (Chekhov), 200–201

Hardy, Thomas, 112–13, 120
Harry (char.), 23–24, 25, 30, 33, 44,
    129–31, 132, 134, 136, 137,
    139
Harvey, William, 69, 76, 184, 186
Health and Human Services Depart-
    ment, U.S., 35
"Heartache" (Chekhov), 60
"Heathen, The" (London), 113–14, 118,
    120–21
Heaven's Coast (Doty), 146
Heidegger, Martin, 195
Hemingway, Ernest, 23–24, 25, 34, 41,
    44, 129–31, 134
Hermann, Nellie, 167, 199

Holocaust, 58
"House of Mapui, The" (London), 115, 117
"How Much Land Does a Man Need?" (Tolstoy), 180–81
Hsi, Steven, 84, 148–49, 151
Human Condition, The (Arendt), 23
Hurry Down Sunshine (Greenberg), 30–31
hypothermia, 116–17

Illness as Metaphor (Sontag), 84, 86
imaginative schema, 111
immunology, 85–86, 117, 177
infectious organisms, 85–86, 117
injury, 94, 95, 104, 125–26, 195–96
    agency and, 89–90, 94–96
    battlefield, 42
    variable connection between pain and, 42–43
    visible, 41–43, 90, 95
intentionality, 25–27, 39–43, 47, 54, 68, 221n, 222n–23n
    visible injuries and, 41–43
    see also objects of inner experience
interaction metaphors, 188–97
    grammatical structure of, 184–85
    substitution metaphors vs., 184–86
International Association for the Study of Pain, 95–96
Internet, 20, 58, 60, 141, 172, 219
In the Land of Pain (Daudet), 18
Isolation in pain, 15, 19, 20, 23–35, 41, 47, 54, 98, 129, 133, 139
    as epoché, 26–27, 29, 98, 106, 130, 138, 142–43, 160, 215, 218, 221n
    from inside, 28–29
    in literature, 23–24, 27–28, 32, 57–58
    in nonfiction, 28–29, 30–31
    of observers, 30–35, 43, 184, 214
    observers' skepticism in, 32–35, 43, 50, 102, 131, 133–34, 137
    ontological divide in, 32–35, 146
    as pain in itself, 67–68

pain medication dosages and, 34–35
shifted perspective in, 25–26, 137–38, 171–72
It's Always Something (Radner), 87

Jamison, Kay Redfield, 96
Johnson, Mark, 110–11, 119
Journey Round My Skull, A (Karinthy), 155
Joyce, James, 17, 65–66, 68–70, 71, 72, 180, 181, 213, 215, 216
Just and Unjust Wars (Walzer), 79

Kahlo, Frida, 17, 104, 105, 156–57, 157, 158, 173–76, 175, 181, 185, 186, 197–98, 198, 200
Karinthy, Frigyes, 154–55, 156, 165
Kings County Hospital, 33–34, 79, 133
knowledge, acquisition of, 45–47, 69, 124, 185, 230n
    mimesis in, 156
    presence of others required for, 152–53
    scientific, 76
    self-, 1331–32, 145–53
    visual perception in, 169
Kuhn, Thomas, 76
Kupferman, Irving, 231n

Lady Chatterley's Lover (Lawrence), 199–200
Lakoff, George, 119
Langer, Susanne, 77, 98, 144–45, 232n
language, 38, 39, 40, 42, 47, 67–68, 125, 139, 154, 194, 210–11, 213–19
    deconstructionist view of, 126
    extension of, 73–77
    force possessed by, 112
    literal vs. metaphorical, 70–72
    as self-extension, 107
    sharable world as anchor of, 88–90
    thoughts influenced by, 73–74

Lawrence, D. H., 199–200
Leg to Stand On, A (Sacks), 28–29
leprosy, 103, 196

Leriche, René, 197
leukemia, 87
Levertov, Denise, 106
Little Deer, The (Kahlo), 174
locked-in syndrome, 60
London, Jack, 160, 178, 200, 215, 218
   anatomic metaphors of, 183–84, 185,
      186, 189–97, 207
   literary agency of, 98, 99–101, 103,
      107, 113–14, 115, 116–17, 118,
      120–21, 124, 128
   projection metaphors of, 135–36, 137,
      139
"Lost on the Steppe" (Tolstoy), 101, 102,
   103, 106, 107, 108, 110, 118, 121
"Love of Life" (London), 183–84
lower back pain, 104

McGill Pain Questionnaire, 13, 80–82,
   81, 83, 158
Madame Bovary (Flaubert), 156
Magic Mountain, The (Mann), 167–69,
   170–72
Maimonides, 75
manic depression, 96
Mann, Thomas, 167–69, 170–72
Man's Search for Meaning (Frankl), 58
Mason (char.), 99–101, 107
"Master and Man" (Tolstoy), 142–45,
   161–63, 180–81
Maupassant, Guy de, 98, 101–3, 104,
     107, 108, 110, 128, 134–35,
     136, 137, 139
Maxwell, James Clerk, 76
Melzack, Ronald, 42–43, 80–82, *81,* 196
Memorial Sloan-Kettering Cancer
   Center, 173
Memory (Kahlo), *105,* 174
Merleau-Ponty, Maurice, 19, 54, 56, 78,
     106, 138, 139–40, 145–46, 153,
     193, 210, 211, 221*n,* 229*n*
metaphors, 13, 15–16, 65–78, 124–26,
   216–19
   aging, 72, 216
   catachretic function of, 73–77, 186
   classification function of, 187

cognitive reach of, 184–87
as conceptual vehicles, 69, 75, 76,
   122, 123
as deviation or necessity, 70–72, 77
filling voids as function of, 73–77
problems of, 125–26
in religion, 75
scientific use of, 69, 76, 184, 186
theorists of, 71, 73–74, 184–85, 232*n*
as tropes, 71, 77
worldmaking and, 68–70, 77–78
migraines, 42, 79–80, 82, 85, 90, 93,
   104, 108, 196
military metaphor, 84–88, 92, 94, 123, 124
Miller, Jonathan, 172, 180, 184, 186
mirror, metaphor of, 16, 129–66
   see also projection metaphors
mirror neurons, 153–57, 230*n*
Mitchell, Joyce, 87
Moore, Lorrie, 129, 131
Morrison, Toni, 96, 146–47, 151, 160–
   61, 218
"Mud Below, The" (Proulx), 97
Munch, Edvard, 11, *12,* 16, 17, 18, 27,
   48, 57–58, 100, 108, 158, 214
myth, 77

Nietzsche, Friedrich, 125–26, 136–37
nitrogen mustard, 86
Nixon, Richard, 87
nominalism, 74

objects of inner experience, 25–27,
   39–43, 45, 46, 68–70, 89
   agency and, 101, 102, 103, 106–7,
     108
   exteriorization enabled by, 40
   projections of aliveness onto, 118–19
   shared, 40, 41, 69–70
   visible injuries as, 41–43
observers of pain, 30–35, 184, 214
   readers as, 100, 101, 103, 107, 109–
     10, 113, 135–36
   skepticism of, 32–35, 43, 50, 102,
     131, 133–34, 137
O'Keeffe, Georgia, 199

"On Being Ill" (Woolf), 28, 57–58
"Open Boat, The" (Crane), 108–110,
    118, 163–64, 215
Otis, Laura, 232n
Our Mutual Friend (Dickens), 201–2

Padfield, Deborah, 177–80, 178, 179
pain:
    body's responses as cause of, 116–17
    chronic, incidence of, 14, 221n
    clinical depression caused by, 37
    congenital and acquired insensitivity
        to, 103, 196
    crisis of, 15, 47, 66, 67–68, 70,
        98–99, 107, 130, 140
    definitions of, 18, 75, 95–96, 104
    everything but itself consumed by, 18,
        19, 26, 37, 75, 104, 108, 213–
        14, 215
    explanation demanded by, 46–47, 93,
        124, 125, 127, 174, 189
    feeling of impending destruction in,
        105–6
    as functioning word, 50, 54–55,
        89–90, 91, 93, 97, 127, 209
    injury equated with, 42, 89, 94–96,
        94, 95, 104, 125–26, 195–96
    of others, alleviation of, 164–65
    phenomenology of, 92–93, 94, 122
    positive side of, 194–97
    prelinguistic state conferred by,
        89–90, 107–8, 209
    resignation to, 37
    sufferer diminished by, 115–16
    varying experience of, 18, 42–43, 95,
        194, 196
    as warning signal, 103–4, 106, 135,
        196–97
pain asymbolia, 227n
pain clinics, 13, 70, 80, 133, 166, 177
pain medication, 42
    addictiveness of, 35
    adequate vs. inadequate doses of,
        34–35, 133–34, 214, 217, 222n
pain thresholds, 43
pain wall, 15, 23, 30–32, 41, 48, 54, 55,
        100, 133, 214

paradigm shifts, 76, 186
paresthesias, 83
pathographies, 85, 87, 200
pathological anatomy, field of, 151–52,
        169–70
Paul D (char.), 146–47, 160
Pears, David, 226n
Peirce, C. S., 136
phagocytes, 85–86
phantom pain, 46, 196
phenomenologists, 25, 26, 40, 221n
Philoctetes (Sophocles), 11, 27
Philosophical Investigations (Wittgen-
        stein), 48, 49–55, 89
photographic collages, 177–80, 178, 179
physicians, 11, 13, 14–15, 42, 58, 70,
        79, 95–96, 116, 127, 154–55,
        172, 180, 213, 214
    inadequate pain medication adminis-
        tered by, 34–35, 133–34, 214,
        217, 222n
    and individual body awareness, 44,
        45
    limited knowledge of, 132
    pain specialists, 80–82
    pathological anatomy field created by,
        151–52, 169–70
    skeptical reactions of, 33–35, 43, 80,
        133
    sympathy lost by, 36–37
physicists, 76
Pinker, Steven, 225n
Portrait of the Artist as a Young Man, A
        (Joyce), 65–66, 68–70
post-herpetic neuralgia, 80
postmodernism, 126
prelinguistic state, 78, 89–90, 91–93,
        91, 107–8, 209
Price, Reynolds, 83–84, 92, 116, 121,
        124, 128
primordial existence, 78
Private Battle, A (Ryan and Ryan), 87
private-language argument, 51–54, 209
private world, 49–55, 56, 57, 209
projection metaphors, 16, 17, 68–69,
        129–66, 174, 180, 197, 207,
        215

abstract entities as, 150
and anatomic metaphors, 197–206
artifacts as, 157–66
boats as, 149, 156, 163–64, 165,
     166
as body extensions, 140, 158,
     163–64
clothing as, 161–63, 166
crows as, 134–35, 136, 137, 139
fellow sufferers and, 141, 145,
     147–49, 154, 165
house as, 160–61, 166
and inaccessibility of body, 150–53
mirror neurons and, 153–57
pain alleviation and, 164–65
responsive world created by, 131,
     137–45
rooster as, 146–47
scavengers as, 130–31, 132, 134, 136,
     137
self-knowledge bestowed by, 131–32,
     145–53
trees as, 143–44, 145, 149–50
validation provided by, 131, 132–37
voices acquired by, 131, 132, 134–35,
     137, 142–44
projections of aliveness, 118–19
Proulx, Annie, 97, 128
psychological pain, 18–19, 95, 96, 214,
     223n
     see also depression; grief
public side of pain, 48–55, 61, 93, 99,
     127, 176
     contexts and behaviors of pain in,
         89–90
     metaphor in, 69–70
     private-language argument and,
         51–54, 209
     private world vs., 49–55, 56, 57, 209

Quintilian, 185

Rachel J (patient), 79–80, 82, 85, 90,
     92, 93, 104, 115, 128, 133
radiation therapy, 87
Radner, Gilda, 87, 128
Ramachandran, V. S., 154

referred pain, 45–46
Remembrance of an Open Wound
     (Kahlo), 174
rhetoric, 70, 72, 73, 74, 87, 125, 215
rheumatoid arthritis, 34, 85, 141
Richards, I. A., 185
Ricoeur, Paul, 71, 185, 232n
Rivera, Diego, 174
Romanticism, 119, 144, 198–99
Roots (Kahlo), 197
Rorty, Richard, 77, 213, 219
Russian formalists, 722, 225n
Ryan, Cornelius and Kathryn, 87
Ryle, Gilbert, 65

Sacks, Oliver, 28–29
Sandy (patient), 85, 141
Sappho, 199
Sartre, Jean-Paul, 152–53, 200, 230n
Scarry, Elaine, 11, 13–14, 16, 32, 33, 38,
     82, 102, 105, 107–8, 112, 118–
     19, 132, 134, 158, 159–60,
     164–65, 195, 207–8, 211, 218
Scream, The (Munch), 11, 12, 18, 48,
     57–58, 100, 108, 214
self-knowledge, 131–32, 145–53
self-mutilation, 133, 165–66
semantics, 74, 225n
"September 1, 1939" (Auden), 185
Sethe (char.), 96, 97, 160–61
Shaw, George Bernard, 85–86, 123
shingles, 80
sickle cell anemia, 33–34, 133
Simon, Carly, 142
"Snows of Kilimanjaro, The" (Heming-
     way), 23–24, 25, 129–31
Solzhenitsyn, Alexander, 27, 41, 87, 92,
     128
Sontag, Susan, 84, 86, 87–88, 123, 167
Sophocles, 11, 27
Stephens, James, 120
string theory, 76
stroke, 25, 60, 148, 150, 188–89, 192
Styron, William, 18–19, 27, 29, 31,
     37–38, 40, 41, 56–57, 67, 68,
     96, 104, 106, 115–16, 177, 215,
     218, 219

substitution metaphors, 73–74
  artifacts as, 181–87
  grammatical structure of, 184–85
  interaction metaphors vs., 184–86
suicide, 29, 58, 106
"Surgical Ward" (Auden), 14, 28, 32, 98
symbol-making, 77
syphilis, tertiary, 18, 83, 141, 148, 149

Takayasu's arteritis, 84
threat, in literary agency, 99–110, 127,
    128, 135–37, 227n
"To Build a Fire" (London), 135–36,
    137, 139, 190–94
"To Fill" (Moore), 129
Tolstoy, Leo, 17, 98, 128, 200, 213, 215,
    216, 218
  anatomic metaphors of, 180–81, 184,
    185
  literary agency of, 101, 102, 103, 106,
    107, 108, 110, 118, 121
  projection metaphors of, 142–45, 151,
    160, 161–63, 166
Torah, 75
Torgerson, Gil, 80–82
Tree of Hope (Kahlo), 174, 197, 198
tuberculosis, 86, 117, 167–69, 170–72,
    182–83, 200–202
Two Fridas, The (Kahlo), 156–57, 157
Tye, Michael, 222n–23n

Unquiet Mind, An (Jamison), 96

visible injuries, 41–43, 90, 95
visualization technique, 176

Wallace, David Foster, 67
Walzer, Michael, 79
war, as agency, 84–88, 124
  cancer and, 86–87, 92, 94, 128
water deprivation, 202–6
Ways of Worldmaking (Goodman), 156
weapon, metaphor of, 16, 79–96, 122–
    23, 174, 177–78
  see also agency, language of
white blood cells, 85–86
"White Silence, The" (London), 99–101,
    103, 107, 116–17, 118
Whole New Life, A (Price), 83–84
Wiman, Christian, 149–50, 151, 165
"Wine on the Desert" (Brand), 202–6
Winning the Chemo Battle (Mitchell), 87
Wit (Edson), 123
Wittgenstein, Ludwig, 19, 48–55, 56,
    57, 61, 69, 74, 89, 126–27, 203,
    209–10, 211, 213, 226n
Woodlanders, The (Hardy), 112–13, 120
Woolf, Virginia, 14, 16, 17, 28, 39,
    57–58, 68, 98, 114, 200
worldmaking, 68–70, 77–78, 108, 132,
    139
World War II, 86
  battlefields of, 42

X-ray, metaphor of, 16, 167–211
  see also anatomic metaphors

Year of Magical Thinking, The (Didion),
    18–19, 20, 59
Yiddish Policemen's Union, The (Cha-
    bon), 217, 218